Veterinary Nursing:

Self-Assessment Questions and Answers Book II

Veterinary Nursing:

Self-Assessment Questions and Answers Book II

J. E. Ouston MA Vet MB MRCVS
Veterinary Surgeon and Lecturer in Veterinary Nursing
Farnborough College of Technology, Hampshire

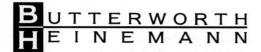

Butterworth-Heinemann
Linacre House, Jordan Hill, Oxford OX2 8DP
A division of Reed Educational and Professional Publishing Ltd

A member of the Reed Elsevier plc group

OXFORD   BOSTON   JOHANNESBURG
MELBOURNE   NEW DELHI   SINGAPORE

First published 1997

© Reed Educational and Professional Publishing Ltd 1997

British Library Cataloguing in Publication Data
A catalogue record for this book is available from the British Library

ISBN 0 7506 3732 3

Typeset by Keyword Typesetting Ltd, Wallington, Surrey
Printed and bound in Great Britain by Biddles Ltd, Guildford and King's Lynn

Contents

Preface   vi

5   General nursing   1
   General nursing   1

6   Diagnostic tests   3
   Diagnostic tests   3

7   Medical nursing   9
   Elementary microbiology   9
   Elementary parasitology   12
   Infectious diseases   15
   Immunity and vaccination   19
   Medical diseases and their nursing   21
   Poisons   24
   Fluid therapy   26

8   Radiography   29
   Radiography   29

9   Surgical nursing   34
   General surgical nursing   34
   Anaesthesia and analgesia   38
   Surgical instruments and equipment   44
   Sterilization and maintenance of an aseptic theatre   46
   Suture materials and suturing   48

10 Obstetrical and paediatric nursing   50
   Obstetrics and paediatrics   50

Answers   55

Preface

The multiple choice format for the Veterinary Nursing Examinations was introduced in 1993. The Royal College of Veterinary Surgeons produced sample papers for the Part I and Part II examinations, but the student nurses I was teaching at the time requested more and more questions in the multiple choice format in order to test their knowledge and practise their exam technique. Over the last few years I have written many multiple choice questions to help train the nurses I teach, and I have received requests for questions from those I am not directly involved with. These books have been compiled in response to these requests, and I hope that they will be of benefit to all nurses as they prepare for the RCVS examinations.

The subjects are presented in the same order as the RCVS Veterinary Nursing syllabus. At the beginning of each subject I have given the number of questions to provide an indication of the amount of time that should be allowed. In the RCVS examinations, each paper consists of 90 questions and students have 90 minutes in which to complete it. Therefore, to practise examination technique, one minute should be allowed for each question. Each question is presented with four possible answers from which the one correct answer has to be selected.

There are six sections in this book. Section 5: General nursing; Section 6: Diagnostic aids, Section 7: Medical nursing; and Section 8: Radiography are all covered in Paper 1 of the RCVS Part II examination. Section 9: Surgical nursing and Section 10: Obstetrical and paediatric nursing form Paper 2.

Sections 1–4 are found in Questions and Answers in Veterinary Nursing: Part I.

When answering multiple choice questions there are a few general tips that should be followed. Always read the question or opening statement carefully, checking for words like not, or untrue. It is easy to lose marks just by not reading the questions properly. If there are calculations in the section you are covering, it may be best to do the other questions first and come back to the calculations. For many people they take longer than one minute, but they carry no more marks than any other question, so it is important that you do not spend too much time on these and so not leave yourself with enough time for the rest of the paper. It is also important not to rush the questions. Pace yourself, ensuring that you answer each question carefully but still allowing yourself sufficient time for a final check of your answers.

The answers for all the questions can be found in a separate section at the end of the book. I have given explanations for the answers, in the hope that this book will also help you to understand the subjects more fully.

JEO

1997

5 General nursing

General nursing

11 Questions

1. **A decubitus ulcer is**
   A   A pressure sore
   B   Ulceration of the mucous membranes
   C   A very deep corneal ulcer
   D   The early stages of gangrene

2. **Higginson's syringe can be used for which of the following?**
   A   Flushing and irrigating the ear canal
   B   Delivering a specific fluid volume via a drip
   C   Giving an enema
   D   Drawing fluid from a chest or abdomen (thoracocentesis or paracentesis)

3. **You have been asked to collect equipment together to catheterize a cat. Which urinary catheter would you select?**
   A   Tiemann's catheter
   B   Jackson's catheter
   C   Dowse's catheter
   D   Foley catheter

4. **If a patient had undergone oesophageal surgery, which method of forced feeding would be most appropriate?**
   A   Orogastric tube
   B   Gastrostomy tube
   C   Nasogastric tube
   D   Pharyngostomy tube

5. **The owners of an elderly dog have asked you for some advice regarding its care. Which of the following would you suggest?**
   A   Restrict fluid availability
   B   Restrict protein in the diet and increase carbohydrate levels
   C   Increase energy levels within the diet
   D   To provide as much exercise as possible, particularly at weekends when the owners are around more.

6. How large is 1 unit French Gauge?
 A   1/4 mm
 B   1/3 mm
 C   1/2 mm
 D   3/4 mm

7. The size of tube you should use for nasogastric intubation of a medium-sized dog is
 A   3–4 FG
 B   4–6 FG
 C   6–8 FG
 D   12 FG

8. The disease which is not associated with older age is
 A   Osteoarthritis
 B   Periodontal disease
 C   Osteochondrosis
 D   Diabetes mellitus

9. Dysphagia is
 A   Difficulty in swallowing
 B   Difficulty in eating
 C   Difficulty in breathing
 D   Difficulty in chewing

10. Prolonged recumbency can lead to several complications. Which is potentially the most serious?
 A   Decubitus ulcers
 B   Hypostatic pneumonia
 C   Joint stiffness
 D   Muscle wastage

11. Constipation in patients can be prevented by the use of
 A   Low fibre diets
 B   Kaolin
 C   High fibre diets
 D   None of the above

The answers are on page 55

6 Diagnostic tests

Diagnostic tests

34 Questions

1. **A centrifuge would be needed in order to carry out which of the following tests?**
   A   Measurement of packed cell volume (PCV)
   B   Haemoglobin estimation
   C   Red blood cell count
   D   Platelet count

2. **A Wintrobe tube can be used for**
   A   Measuring glucose concentrations
   B   Measuring PCV
   C   Collecting urine output
   D   Giving blood

3. **Dehydration is characterized by**
   A   Increased PCV and decreased plasma protein level
   B   Decreased PCV and decreased plasma protein level
   C   Decreased PCV and increased plasma protein level
   D   Increased PCV and increased plasma protein level

4. **Variation in erythrocyte size on a blood smear is called**
   A   Spherocytosis
   B   Poikilocytosis
   C   Anisocytosis
   D   Anisochromasia

5. **When present in urine, which substance can mask a positive glucose reaction on urine dipsticks?**
   A   Ketones
   B   Blood
   C   Penicillin
   D   Ascorbic acid

6. **A 10-year-old dog with chronic renal failure has a blood urea nitrogen of 90 mg/dl and a serum creatinine level of 4.0 mg/dl. The specific gravity of urine from this dog is most likely to be**
   A   Between 1.020 and 1.040
   B   Between 1.006 and 1.025
   C   Less than 1.006
   D   Between 1.030 and 1.055

7. **A cat is presented with pinpoint haemorrhages on the skin and mucous membranes. What is the most likely haematological abnormality?**
   A   Increased packed cell volume
   B   Decreased PCV
   C   Increased platelet count
   D   Decreased platelet count

8. **Severe parasitism can result in which of the following changes in the white blood cell picture?**
   A   Eosinophilia
   B   Neutrophilia
   C   Lymphocytosis
   D   Monocytosis

9. **The normal packed cell volume (PCV) for a cat expressed as a percentage is**
   A   10–15
   B   16–23
   C   24–45
   D   46–58

10. **A blood smear for a differential white blood cell count should be stained using which of the following?**
    A   Leishman's stain
    B   Gram's stain
    C   Lugol's iodine
    D   New methylene blue

11. **In a complete blood count, a left shift refers to**
    A   Movement of the microscope slide to the left
    B   Decreased numbers of platelets
    C   An abundance of immature white blood cell forms
    D   Increased numbers of nucleated red blood cells

12. **Increased serum amylase and lipase activities usually suggest**
    A   Liver disease
    B   Kidney disease
    C   Intestinal disease
    D   Pancreatic disease

13. **Where are urinary casts produced in the urinary tract?**
    A   Kidney tubules
    B   Ureter
    C   Bladder
    D   Urethra

14. **The method that can be used to test for the presence of protein in urine is**
    A   Hay's test
    B   Copper sulphate test
    C   Fouchet's test
    D   Benedict's reagent

15. **What is the normal red blood cell count for a dog?**
    A 6–$18 \times 10^9/l$
    B 5.5–$8.5 \times 10^9/l$
    C 5.5–$8.5 \times 10^{12}/l$
    D 6–$18 \times 10^{12}/l$

16. **The white blood cells which usually make up 5% of the differential count are**
    A   Neutrophils
    B   Basophils
    C   Lymphocytes
    D   Monocytes

17. **The reason white blood cell diluting fluid contains acetic acid is**
    A   To lyse the red blood cells
    B   To lyse the white blood cells
    C   To make the white blood cells more easily visible under the microscope
    D   To suspend the cells

18. **In order to determine a differential white blood cell count, what is the minimum number of white blood cells that should be counted?**
    A   50
    B   100
    C   200
    D   500

19. **The enzyme or biochemical parameter which gives most information about damage to liver cells is**
    A   ALT
    B   AST
    C   Cholesterol
    D   Bilirubin

20. **When examining faecal smears, which stain is used to identify undigested fats?**
    A   Alcoholic Sudan III
    B   Lugol's iodine
    C   Eosin
    D   New methylene blue

21. **Some Dalmatians suffer from a hereditary condition in which they are prone to crystalluria. Which crystal is found in the urine from these animals?**
    A   Urate
    B   Calcium oxalate
    C   Struvite (triple phosphate)
    D   Cystine

22. **Urine intended for bacterial studies should be preserved using**
    A   Toluene
    B   Formalin
    C   Thymol
    D   Boric acid

23. **If you had collected a urine sample by catheterizing a patient, which of the following would indicate clinical disease?**
    A   Mucus
    B   Spermatozoa
    C   White cell casts
    D   Transitional epithelial cells

24. **If you are staining a blood smear with Leishman's stain, how long should you leave the undiluted stain on the smear?**
    A   2 minutes
    B   5 minutes
    C   10 minutes
    D   20 minutes

25. How is the total magnification of a microscope calculated?
A   Eyepiece magnification + Objective magnification
B   Eyepiece magnification × Objective magnification
C   Eyepiece magnification ÷ Objective magnification
D   Eyepiece magnification − Objective magnification

26. The stain used to examine fungi is
A   Gram's stain
B   Lactophenol cotton blue
C   Wright's stain
D   Iodine

27. What does a colorimeter measure?
A   The amount of light emitted by a coloured solution
B   The concentration of any substance in solution
C   The amount of light absorbed by a coloured solution
D   The different colours of light that will pass through a particular solution

28. Before drawing off serum, a blood sample should be allowed to clot for at least
A   10 minutes
B   30 minutes
C   1 hour
D   2 hours

29. The bacterium that needs to be stained using the Ziehl–Neelsen staining technique is
A   *Clostridium tetani*
B   Streptococcus
C   Salmonella
D   *Mycobacterium tuberculosis*

30. A supravital staining technique has to be used to identify which of the following cell types?
A   Red blood cells
B   Platelets
C   Neutrophils
D   Reticulocytes

31. **Which abnormal constituent would you find in the urine of a dog suffering from obstructive jaundice?**
    A   Protein
    B   Blood
    C   Bilirubin
    D   Fatty casts

32. **The bacteria which would appear as Gram-negative rods under the light microscope are**
    A   Streptococci
    B   Staphylococci
    C   *Clostridium tetani*
    D   *Escherichia coli*

33. **The McKenzie brush technique used as a diagnostic method for**
    A   Ringworm
    B   Sarcoptic mange
    C   Staphylococcal dermatitis
    D   Lice infestations

34. **Which urinary crystals are usually hexagonal in appearance?**
    A   Struvite (ammonium triple phosphate)
    B   Urate
    C   Cystine
    D   Calcium oxalate

The answers are on page 58

7 Medical nursing

Elementary microbiology

13 Questions

1. **The difference between Gram-negative and Gram-positive bacteria is**
   A Gram-negative bacteria do not have flagella
   B Gram-positive bacteria have an extra cell wall layer
   C Gram-negative bacteria have an extra cell wall layer
   D Gram-negative bacteria are not pathogenic

2. **Bacteria reproduce in which of the following ways?**
   A Conjugation
   B Spore formation
   C Simple binary fission
   D Mitosis

3. **Structural components of all viruses include**
   A A capsule, cell wall and a cell membrane
   B A cell wall, a cytoplasmic membrane and nucleic acid
   C A protein capsid and nucleic acid
   D An envelope, DNA, RNA and a cell wall

4. **The bacterium which can form spores is**
   A *Staphylococcus aureus*
   B *Clostridium tetani*
   C *Escherichia coli*
   D *Bordetella bronchiseptica*

5. **Which statement is true about exotoxins?**
   A They are very heat stable
   B They are not usually very toxic
   C They are produced by Gram-positive bacteria
   D They are only released when the bacterium dies

6. **Wood's lamp examination will cause which fungal species to fluoresce in some cases?**
   A Trichophyton
   B Aspergillus
   C Microsporum
   D Candida

7. **The type of medium used to culture fungi is**
   - A Selenite broth
   - B Sabouraud's medium
   - C McConkey agar
   - D Desoxycholate citrate agar

8. **Which of the following is a selective medium?**
   - A Nutrient agar
   - B Chocolate agar
   - C Selenite broth
   - D Blood agar

9. **Anaerobic conditions are required to grow which type of bacteria?**
   - A Streptococci
   - B *Escherichia coli*
   - C Leptospira
   - D Clostridia

10. **An example of a pathogenic yeast is**
    - A Aspergillus
    - B Trichophyton
    - C Candida
    - D Microsporum

11. **What size (roughly) are viruses?**
    - A Nanometres, nm (1×10^{-9}m)
    - B Micrometres, μm (1×10^{-6}m)
    - C Picometres, pm (1×10^{-12}m)
    - D Millimetres, mm (1×10^{-3}m)

12. **The term 'facultative anaerobe' is used to describe**
    - A A bacterium that has an absolute requirement for oxygen
    - B A bacterium that grows optimally without oxygen
    - C A bacterium that can grow in the absence of oxygen but grows better when oxygen is present
    - D A bacterium that grows best in the presence of tiny quantities of oxygen

13. **Dermatophyte test medium (DTM) changes colour if fungi are cultured on its surface. What colour does it turn?**
    A   Orange
    B   Yellow
    C   Red
    D   Brown

The answers are on page 67

Elementary parasitology

16 Questions

1. **A dog is presented at the surgery with alopecia around the eyes and muzzle without obvious pruritus. Which mite do you suspect?**
    A   *Otodectes cynotis*
    B   *Demodex canis*
    C   *Sarcoptes scabiei*
    D   *Cheyletiella yasguri*

2. **The larval stage of *Toxocara canis* which is infective is**
    A L_4
    B L_3
    C L_2
    D L_1

3. **What is the proper name of the hookworm?**
    A   *Uncinaria stenocephala*
    B   *Trichuris vulpis*
    C   *Toxascaris leonina*
    D   *Oslerus osleri*

4. **Lice can be divided into two types, sucking and biting. Which of the following is a sucking louse?**
    A   *Ctenocephalides felis*
    B   *Linognathus setosus*
    C   *Trichodectes canis*
    D   *Felicola subrostratus*

5. ***Trombicula autumnalis* can cause clinical disease in some cats and dogs. Which stage of its life cycle is parasitic?**
    A   Larva
    B   Nymph
    C   Adult
    D   All of the above

6. **An intermediate host is always required by which of the following parasites?**
    A   *Toxocara canis*
    B   *Toxoplasma gondii*
    C   *Toxascaris leonina*
    D   *Taenia hydatigena*

7. **The parasite which typically causes intense pruritus and crusting of the ear tips is**
   A   *Demodex canis*
   B   *Trichodectes canis*
   C   *Cheyletiella yasguri*
   D   *Sarcoptes scabiei*

8. **You are performing faecal flotation on the faeces from a dog, and find a lemon-shaped egg with a plug at each end. Which worm is the dog infested with?**
   A   *Trichuris vulpis*
   B   *Uncinaria stenocephala*
   C   *Toxocara canis*
   D   *Toxascaris leonina*

9. **The eggs of which parasite are glued to the hair shafts of its host?**
   A   *Ctenocephalides felis*
   B   *Sarcoptes scabiei*
   C   *Otodectes cynotis*
   D   *Linognathus setosus*

10. **Toxoplasma can be transmitted from one host to another via all of the following routes except**
    A   Via meat from an intermediate host containing the organism
    B   Via the milk from queen to kitten
    C   Via food contaminated by cat faeces
    D   Via the placenta and afterbirths of aborted lambs

11. **The term which describes infestation by dipteran larvae is**
    A   Mydriasis
    B   Meiosis
    C   Myiasis
    D   Miosis

12. **The whipworm of dogs is**
    A   *Aelurostrongylus abstrusus*
    B   *Oslerus osleri*
    C   *Trichuris vulpis*
    D   *Uncinaria stenocephala*

13. **Pruritus and excessive epidermal scaling can be produced by which non-burrowing mite?**
    A *Cheyletiella*
    B *Notoedres*
    C *Sarcoptes*
    D *Otodectes*

14. **The parasite that reproduces asexually is**
    A *Toxocara cati*
    B *Taenia hydatigena*
    C *Ixodes ricinus*
    D *Felicola subrostratus*

15. **Visceral Larva Migrans in man is caused by which parasite?**
    A Toxocara species
    B *Toxascaris leoninum*
    C *Toxoplasma gondii*
    D *Echinococcus granulosus*

16. **A paratenic host is best defined by which of the following statements?**
    A The host in which a parasite has to undergo part of its life cycle before it can reinfest the final host
    B A host which carries an organism, and sheds it intermittently
    C The animal in which the adult or reproductive phase of the parasite occurs
    D A host which carries an immature parasite in its tissues. It has to be eaten by the final host for the parasite to complete its life cycle

The answers are on page 71

Infectious diseases

19 Questions

1. **The cause of feline infectious anaemia is**
   A   Feline leukaemia virus
   B   Coronavirus
   C   Parvovirus
   D   *Haemobartonella felis*

2. **'Blue eye' is a complication encountered in dogs vaccinated with**
   A   Live canine distemper vaccine
   B   Inactivated canine adenovirus-1 vaccine
   C   Live canine adenovirus-1 vaccine
   D   Leptospira vaccine

3. **You test a 2-year-old clinically normal cat from a single-cat household for feline leukaemia virus infection with an in-house test kit. The result of the test is positive. What is the most appropriate advice for the owner?**
   A   Isolate the cat and retest in two to three months
   B   Euthanase the cat before it develops full-blown infection
   C   The result was probably inaccurate
   D   Isolate the cat, but do not bother to retest, as the second test is likely to be positive

4. **The incubation period for parvovirus in dogs is**
   A   2–3 days
   B   3–5 days
   C   5–7 days
   D   Over a week

5. **Which of the following organisms can become latent after an initial infection?**
   A   Feline parvovirus
   B   Canine adenovirus-1
   C   Feline herpes virus 1
   D   *Bordetella bronchiseptica*

6. **In samples of which bodily fluids might you find leptospira organisms in an infected animal?**
   A   Gut secretions and faeces
   B   Blood
   C   Urine
   D   Both blood and urine

7. **Chlamydia infection in a cat can be diagnosed using which diagnostic technique?**
    A CITE test
    B Microscopy of conjunctival scraping
    C Haematology
    D Microscopic examination of lacrimal fluid

8. **What is a fomite?**
    A Another host that carries an organism in which the organism undergoes part of its life cycle
    B An inanimate object that comes into contact with an infected animal, becomes contaminated, and then comes into contact with a non-infected animal.
    C Another host that carries the organism and can shed it at any time
    D Another host that carries the organism and has to be eaten to pass on the infection

9. ***Haemobartonella felis* is thought to be carried by fleas. Which term best describes the way the fleas act as carriers?**
    A Biological vector
    B Intermediate host
    C Transport host
    D Paratenic host

10. **Which set of clinical signs most closely describes infection in the dog by canine adenovirus-1?**
    A Acute myocarditis or gastro-enteritis
    B One of several syndromes including oculonasal discharges, pharyngitis, hyperkeratosis of pads and nose, nervous signs
    C Acute pyrexia, petechial haemorrhages on gums, hepatic enlargement, possible neurological signs, collapse and death
    D Dry hacking cough, retching, gagging and occasional serous nasal and ocular discharges

11. **The disease which is zoonotic is**
    A Canine parvovirus
    B Canine distemper
    C Canine hepatitis
    D Leptospirosis

12. **What is a saprophyte?**
    A   An organism that lives on a larger organism and causes disease
    B   An organism that lives on dead organic matter
    C   An organism that benefits its host
    D   An organism that causes no harm or good to its host

13. **Viral diseases can be positively diagnosed in the live animal using which of the following methods?**
    A   Histology
    B   Clinical signs
    C   Rising antibody titre
    D   A single measurement of serum antibody levels

14. **All of the following statements are true about feline infectious peritonitis except**
    A   The mode of transmission is not well understood
    B   It can produce two forms of the disease, a wet and a dry form
    C   The organism is resistant to many disinfectants, and can remain in the environment for long periods of time
    D   The fluid produced in the wet form is high in protein

15. **Canine parvovirus is thought to have evolved from which other infectious virus?**
    A   Canine distemper virus
    B   Feline influenza virus
    C   Feline panleucopaenia virus
    D   Canine herpes virus

16. **The feline infectious agent that causes chronic stomatitis and gingivitis is**
    A   *Chlamydia psittaci*
    B   *Haemobartonella felis*
    C   Feline calici virus
    D   Coronavirus

17. Which organism can last in the environment for up to a year?
A   Canine parvovirus
B   Canine distemper virus
C   Canine adenovirus
D   *Leptospira icterohaemorrhagiae*

18. For barrier nursing all of the following statements are true except
A   Nurses should wear waterproof aprons, gloves and boots
B   They should treat isolated cases before the remainder of the in-patients
C   Animals in isolation should have their own sets of food bowls, cleaning utensils, grooming equipment and bedding
D   Animals with the same disease condition can be placed together in an isolation ward

19. If an unvaccinated cat is exposed to Feline leukaemia virus for the first time, it is most likely to lead to persistent infection if the cat is
A   Over four months of age
B   Six to eight weeks of age
C   Elderly
D   A neonate

The answers are on page 75

Immunity and vaccination

8 Questions

1. **Cellular immunity involves the activities of which cells?**
   A   B-cells, mast cells and T-cells
   B   Neutrophils, mast cells and histiocytes
   C   Monocytes and T-cells
   D   Mast cells, monocytes and histiocytes

2. **Mature antibody-producing cells are called**
   A   Immunoblasts
   B   T-cells
   C   B-cells
   D   Neutrophils

3. **Animals are not routinely vaccinated before they reach eight to nine weeks of age because**
   A   Their immune system is too poorly developed to be able to respond
   B   There may still be maternal antibodies within the plasma
   C   There may still be maternal T- and B-cells within the plasma
   D   The dose of the vaccine would be too great, and the animals would develop clinical signs

4. **What does a toxoid contain?**
   A   Antigen from micro-organism
   B   Antibodies to a toxin
   C   Antigen from a toxin
   D   Antibodies to a micro-organism

5. **The canine infectious disease which is always protected against with a dead vaccine is**
   A   Parvovirus
   B   Distemper
   C   Infectious canine hepatitis
   D   Leptospirosis

6. **Which of the following is true about dead vaccines?**
   A   Only one dose is needed for good protection
   B   They are less long lasting in effect than live vaccines
   C   They are less safe than live vaccines
   D   Most vaccines currently used are dead vaccines

7. **Live attenuated vaccines should be stored at what temperature?**
   A $< +2°C$
   B $+2$ to $+8°C$
   C $+5$ to $+10°C$
   D $+10$ to $+15°C$

8. **The release of interferon is stimulated by**
   A   Infection with a virus
   B   Infection with bacteria
   C   Parasitic infestation
   D   Any of the above

The answers are on page 81

Medical diseases and their nursing

18 Questions

1. **For which of the following conditions would you advise a diet containing restricted levels of protein and sodium?**
   A Colitis
   B Feline urologic syndrome
   C Food allergy
   D Renal disease

2. **A hyperthyroid cat would show all of these clinical signs except**
   A Bradycardia
   B Weight loss
   C Heat intolerance
   D Mild diarrhoea

3. **The cardiac disease which is congenital is**
   A Endocardiosis
   B Cardiomyopathy
   C Myocarditis
   D Persistent right aortic arch

4. **The clinical sign that is not typically associated with small intestinal diarrhoea is**
   A Tenesmus
   B Weight loss
   C Polyphagia
   D Borborygmi

5. **A patient could develop keto-acidosis in which of the following conditions?**
   A Diabetes insipidus
   B Hyperthyroidism
   C Hypothyroidism
   D Diabetes mellitus

6. **An animal suffering from left-sided heart failure would show which of the following signs?**
   A Ascites
   B Right-sided cardiac enlargement
   C Pulmonary oedema leading to a cough
   D Jugular pulse

7. **Furunculosis is a severe example of which skin disease?**
   A   Pyoderma
   B   Seborrhoea
   C   Alopecia
   D   Hormonal disease

8. **The insulin with the longest duration of action is**
   A   Insuvet neutral
   B   Caninsulin
   C   Insuvet protamine zinc
   D   Insuvet lente

9. **Which of the following dietary changes is beneficial in patients with cardiac disease?**
   A   Increase in protein
   B   Increase in digestibility
   C   Decrease in salt
   D   Increase in carbohydrate

10. **Animals which are jaundiced show yellow discoloration of the mucous membranes and sclera. What can cause jaundice?**
    A   Excess red blood cell destruction
    B   Bile duct obstruction
    C   Liver disease
    D   All of the above

11. **Arterial blood pressure is at its maximum during which part of the cardiac cycle?**
    A   Atrial systole
    B   Atrial diastole
    C   Ventricular diastole
    D   Ventricular systole

12. **Hepatic encephalopathy is seen in cases of chronic liver disease due to**
    A   The build up of urea within the circulation
    B   The lack of plasma proteins
    C   Excess bilirubin within the blood stream
    D   The toxic effects of ammonia within the blood stream

13. Which bone condition is associated with chronic renal failure?
A   Marie's disease (chronic pulmonary osteoarthropathy)
B   Rubber jaw (secondary hyperparathyroidism)
C   Lion jaw (craniomandibular osteopathy)
D   Barlow's disease (metaphyseal osteopathy)

14. Food allergies can be diagnosed by
A   Intradermal testing
B   Restriction diets
C   Using antihistamines
D   All of the above

15. Calcium levels within the body are regulated by which hormones?
A   Thyroid hormones
B   Glucocorticoids and mineralocorticoids
C   Insulin and glucagon
D   Parathyroid hormone and calcitonin

16. The management of a fitting animal might include the use of which drug?
A   Phenyl propanolamine
B   Pentobarbitone
C   Prednisolone
D   Phenylbutazone

17. The hormone released by the kidney when blood pressure falls is
A   Erythropoietin
B   Aldosterone
C   Angiotensin
D   Renin

18. Which cardiac disease results in the development of nodules on the cusps of the heart valves, which prevents them opening and closing normally, and is the most common cause of congestive heart failure in the dog?
A   Endocarditis
B   Pericardial effusions
C   Endocardiosis
D   Myocarditis

The answers are on page 84

Poisons

8 Questions

1. **The specific antidote which can be given to an animal suspected of having been poisoned with lead is**
    A   Sodium calcium edetate in saline solution
    B   Ethanol + sodium bicarbonate
    C   Atropine sulphate
    D   Acetyl cysteine

2. **Animals with ethylene glycol poisoning often develop which crystal within their urine?**
    A   Cystine
    B   Urate
    C   Calcium oxalate
    D   Struvite (ammonium triple phosphate)

3. **Chronic lead poisoning leads to the development of which of the following clinical signs?**
    A   Vomiting and diarrhoea
    B   Acute interstitial pneumonia
    C   Abnormal pigmentation of the hair
    D   Nervous signs

4. **The pesticide with an anaesthetic action, which causes a dramatic drop in body temperature and leads to hypothermia and death is**
    A   Sodium chlorate
    B   Paraquat
    C   Metaldehyde
    D   Alphachloralose

5. **If an animal is suspected to have been poisoned by paracetamol, which antidote can be used?**
    A   Sodium calcium edetate in saline solution
    B   Ethanol and sodium bicarbonate
    C   Atropine sulphate
    D   Acetyl cysteine

6. **Vomiting should not be induced in cases of which type of poisoning?**
    A   Ingestion of bleach
    B   Phenol ingestion
    C   Ingestion of petroleum products
    D   All of the above

7. **For what purpose is warfarin used legally?**
   A   Insecticide
   B   Slugbait
   C   Rodenticide
   D   Herbicide

8. **Some poisons cause a change in haemoglobin which leads to a colour change in the animal's blood. Which of the following poisons does this?**
   A   Carbon monoxide
   B   Sodium chlorate
   C   Paracetamol
   D   All of the above

The answers are on page 91

Fluid therapy

1. **A 12.5-kg mongrel has been vomiting for 3 days and is estimated to be 8% dehydrated. What approximate fluid volume should you give to rehydrate this dog?**
    A   500 ml
    B   1000 ml
    C   2000 ml
    D   2240 ml

2. **Which of the following solutions would you give intravenously to maintain an animal once it had been rehydrated?**
    A   Hartmann's solution
    B   Plasma
    C   5% dextrose
    D   0.18% sodium chloride, 4% dextrose (1/5 normal saline)

3. **If you wished to maintain a 36-kg dog on a drip, and you needed to give 2160 ml over 24 hours, how fast would you set the drip? (Assume that 1 ml = 20 drops)**
    A   1 drop per second
    B   1 drop every 2 seconds
    C   1 drop every 3 seconds
    D   2 drops per second

4. **Sodium bicarbonate should not be given with which of the following fluids?**
    A   Hartmann's
    B   Normal saline
    C   5% dextrose
    D   0.18% sodium chloride, 4% dextrose

5. **Over-infusion of a patient with intravenous fluids could lead to**
    A   The development of renal failure
    B   The development of oedema
    C   A fall in central venous pressure
    D   The development of hepatic failure

6. **The type of body water which makes up about 5% of the animal's total body weight is**
   A   Intracellular fluid
   B   Extracellular fluid
   C   Plasma
   D   Synovial fluid

7. **Which of the following conditions would result in a primary water deficit?**
   A   Unconsciousness
   B   Vomiting
   C   Diarrhoea
   D   Burns

8. **The anticoagulant which is used when collecting blood for blood transfusions is**
   A   Acid citrate dextrose (ACD)
   B   Heparin
   C   EDTA
   D   Fluoride oxalate

9. **Central venous pressure provides an indication of the state of an animal's circulation. What is normal central venous pressure in small animals?**
   A   3–7 cm water
   B   150–160 mm water
   C   3–7 mmHg
   D   150–160 mmHg

10. **All the following solutions are isotonic except**
    A   0.9% sodium chloride
    B   5% dextrose
    C   0.18% sodium chloride, 4% dextrose
    D   1.8% sodium chloride

11. **If an animal was suffering from chronic diarrhoea, which would be the most appropriate fluid to use for rehydration?**
    A   Normal saline
    B   5% dextrose
    C   Hartmann's solution
    D   0.18% sodium chloride, 4% dextrose

12. **A 4-kg cat normally has a PCV of 37%, but has become dehydrated and now has a PCV of 44%. How much fluid does it require for rehydration?**
    A   140 ml
    B   200 ml
    C   240 ml
    D   280 ml

13. **In which of the following cases might you need to supplement potassium in the drip?**
    A   An anorexic cat being maintained on intravenous fluids
    B   A pup with acute parvovirus infection
    C   A young adult dog which requires an enterotomy to remove a golf ball
    D   An older dog with a gastric torsion

The answers are on page 93

8 Radiography

Radiography

24 Questions

1. **The grid factor for a grid depends on which of the following?**
   A   Grid ratio
   B   The number of lines per inch
   C   The thickness of the lines
   D   All of the above

2. **Scattered radiation is produced due to the**
   A   Photoelectric effect
   B   Compton effect
   C   Piezo-electric effect
   D   Reflection of X-rays

3. **A 20-kg dog's metacarpal is radiographed using the following exposure factors: FFD = 70 cm, kV = 45 kV, mA = 20 mA, Time = 0.3 sec**
   What are the new exposure factors if the time is increased to 0.4 sec?
   A   FFD = 70 cm, kV = 40 kV, mA = 20 mA
   B   FFD = 70 cm, kV = 45 kV, mA = 15 mA
   C   FFD = 75 cm, kV = 45 kV, mA = 20 mA
   D   FFD = 70 cm, kV = 45 kV, mA = 27 mA

4. **In which part of the X-ray film are the radiation sensitive grains found?**
   A   Supercoat
   B   Subbing layer
   C   Emulsion
   D   Base

5. **Altering which exposure factor will affect the quality of the X-ray beam produced?**
   A   mA
   B   Time
   C   Focal–film distance
   D   kV

6. **The absorption of X-rays by a tissue depends on which of the following?**
   A   Its atomic number
   B   The density of the tissue
   C   The thickness of the tissue
   D   All of the above

7. **The processing sequence for a radiograph is development, fixing and washing. What takes place in the fixer?**
   A   Exposed silver grains are washed off the film
   B   Unexposed silver bromide grains are reduced to metallic silver
   C   Exposed silver bromide grains are reduced to metallic silver
   D   Unexposed silver bromide grains are washed off the film

8. **Which type of contrast medium would be suitable for use in a myelogram?**
   A   High osmolar, ionic water-soluble iodine preparation
   B   Low osmolar, ionic water-soluble iodine preparation
   C   Low osmolar, non-ionic water-soluble iodine preparation
   D   Barium compound

9. **The maximum dose of radiation a member of the general public (over 18) may legally receive to the whole body in a year is**
   A   No dose at all
   B   5 mSv
   C   15 mSv
   D   50 mSv

10. **The use of X-rays in practice is controlled by which piece of legislation?**
   A   Health & Safety at Work Act
   B   COSHH Regulations
   C   Guidance Notes for the Protection of Persons against Ionising Radiations arising from Veterinary Use
   D   Ionising Radiation Regulations 1985

11. **If you examined a radiograph that had been overexposed, how would it appear?**
    A 'Soot and whitewash' film — white subject, dark background, with no internal detail visible
    B Black background, subject detail too dark — a flat film lacking contrast
    C Subject pale, background grey and fails the 'finger test'
    D One area of the radiograph black — generally unrelated to the position of the primary beam

12. **If the distance between the effective focal spot and the object being radiographed is trebled, by how much should you increase the exposure factors to maintain the same radiographic density?**
    A Increase mAs by 3 times
    B Increase kV by 3 times
    C Increase mAs by 9 times
    D Increase kV by 9 times

13. **All of the following are properties of X-rays except**
    A They travel in straight lines
    B They blacken photographic emulsion
    C They can penetrate all materials to some degree
    D They can be reflected by some materials

14. **Which statement is true about different types of grid?**
    A Potter–Bucky is a stationary grid
    B Parallel grids can result in grid cut-off at the edge of the radiograph
    C Focused and pseudo-focused grids are the same type of grid
    D For all types of grid, the exposure factors needed are lower than without the grid

15. **Heat is lost in the rotating anode X-ray tube head by**
    A Conduction through copper
    B Convection through air
    C Radiation through the vacuum
    D Evaporation

16. **There is a rectifier within the X-ray tube head. Why is this needed?**
    A   To change alternating current into direct current
    B   To reduce the voltage to the filament from 240 V to 10 V
    C   To increase the voltage between the anode and cathode from 240 V to 40–80 kV
    D   To prevent fluctuations in the voltage from the mains

17. **If you were developing non-screen film manually, how much longer would you leave the film in the developer compared with screen film?**
    A   Double the normal developing time
    B   Increase by 2 minutes
    C   Increase by 1 minute
    D   Increase by 30 seconds

18. **A dog is radiographed using the following exposure factors: kV = 70 kV, mA = 20 mA, time = 0.2 sec, FFD = 70 cm. You want to introduce a grid with grid factor 4. Which of the following settings could you use?**
    A   kV = 70 kV, mA = 40 mA, time = 0.2 sec, FFD = 70 cm
    B   kV = 80 kV, mA = 20 mA, time = 0.2 sec, FFD = 70 cm
    C   kV = 80 kV, mA = 40 mA, time = 0.2 sec, FFD = 70 cm
    D   kV = 70 kV, mA = 40 mA, time = 0.4 sec, FFD = 80 cm

19. **The radius of the controlled area from the X-ray tube head when used in an unconfined area is**
    A   1 m
    B   2 m
    C   3 m
    D   4 m

20. **By how much does the average lead apron decrease the primary beam?**
    A   Total block of the primary beam
    B   Decreases it by half
    C   Decreases it by three-quarters
    D   Does not really decrease it at all

21. The production of scattered radiation can be reduced by doing all of the following except
A   Compress the part being radiographed
B   Collimate the beam
C   Use a grid
D   Use a lead-backed cassette

22. The statement about screens which is incorrect is
A   Radiation causes crystals in the screens to fluoresce
B   Screens mean that higher exposure factors are required
C   Screens reduce the definition of the radiograph
D   Screen crystals can be made of calcium tungstate

23. There is an aluminium filter incorporated into the window of the X-ray tube head. What is its function?
A   To absorb X-ray beams leaving the tube head at the wrong angle
B   To absorb any low energy X-rays
C   To prevent light getting into the X-ray tube head
D   To absorb heat

24. Developer solutions should be kept in a tank with the lid on
A   To prevent evaporation
B   To prevent contamination with dust
C   To prevent oxidation of the developer chemicals
D   To prevent inhalation of the developer chemicals during times other than processing

The answers are on page 97

9 Surgical nursing

General surgical nursing

20 Questions

1. **All of the following are laparotomy approaches except**
   A   Pararectal
   B   Paracostal
   C   Sublumbar
   D   Paracentesis

2. **After luxation and replacement of which joint would you use an Ehmer sling?**
   A   Stifle
   B   Elbow
   C   Shoulder
   D   Hip

3. **Concerning shock, which statement is the least accurate?**
   A   Shock is a maldistribution of blood flow, causing decreased delivery of oxygen to tissues
   B   Shock should be considered an emergency situation warranting immediate treatment
   C   Shock causes a marked parasympathetic response
   D   Shock can be caused by haemorrhage, severe stress, infection or anaphylaxis

4. **A gastropexy might be indicated in the management of which condition?**
   A   Gastric foreign body
   B   Gastric neoplasia
   C   Gastric torsion
   D   Haemorrhagic gastro-enteritis

5. **Which of the following investigative techniques would provide most information about a lump that was suspected of being a tumour?**
   A   Wedge biopsy
   B   Needle biopsy
   C   Needle aspirate
   D   Exfoliative cytology

6. **The statement about glaucoma that is untrue is**
   A Drainage of aqueous humour is prevented
   B Glaucoma can be inherited
   C Intra-ocular pressure is decreased
   D Left untreated it can lead to permanent retinal damage

7. **In which of the following breeds would you find an increased incidence of tracheal collapse?**
   A Great Dane
   B Labrador
   C Cocker Spaniel
   D Yorkshire Terrier

8. **The condition which could be an indication for performing a urethrostomy in a male animal is**
   A Ruptured bladder
   B Hydronephrosis
   C Urethral calculi
   D Ectopic ureter

9. **Which chemicals are natural inflammatory mediators?**
   A Histamine and prostaglandins
   B Glucocorticoids
   C Adrenaline and noradrenaline
   D All of the above

10. **A transverse fracture of a long bone could be repaired using which of the following techniques?**
    A Cast
    B Plate
    C Intramedullary pin
    D Splint

11. **Animals with lymphosarcoma are most commonly treated using which type of tumour therapy?**
    A Chemotherapy
    B Radiotherapy
    C Surgery
    D Radioactive isotopes

12. **Fracture disease is the term used to describe**
    A   Osteomyelitis
    B   Malunion
    C   Weakening of a bone as a repair device takes all the strain
    D   Electrolysis of a bone due to implants of different metals being used together

13. **If you were on your own dealing with a suspected gastric torsion and had already called the veterinary surgeon, what would you do next?**
    A   Radiograph the abdomen
    B   Trocharize the abdomen using an 18 g needle
    C   Attempt to pass a stomach tube
    D   Operate immediately

14. **All the following tumours affect bone and connective tissue. Which is benign?**
    A   Osteosarcoma
    B   Chondrosarcoma
    C   Osteochondroma
    D   Fibrosarcoma

15. **If liquid nitrogen is being used for cryotherapy, what minimum temperature is reached?**
    A $-20°C$
    B $-40°C$
    C $-100°C$
    D $-150°C$

16. **Cataracts affect which part of the eye?**
    A   Aqueous humour
    B   Lens
    C   Cornea
    D   Retina

17. **Gangrene is**
    A   Formation of an abscess
    B   Mineralization and the deposition of calcium
    C   Sloughing of dead tissues
    D   Death of tissues, with or without bacterial invasion

18. If an animal is suffering from keratitis, which part of the eye is inflamed?
A   Cornea
B   Sclera
C   Conjunctiva
D   Eyelids

19. Which intramedullary pin is often used in pairs for the repair of epiphyseal fractures?
A   Steinmann pin
B   Rush pin
C   Kuntscher nail
D   Any of the above

20. A drain could be used in which of the following situations?
A   A shallow wound healing by second intention
B   A deep wound in which dead space has been produced by the surgical removal of some tissue
C   A small surgical wound healing by first intention
D   A cystotomy

The answers are on page 105

Anaesthesia and analgesia

1. **The premedicant agent which has significant analgesic effects is**
   A   Acepromazine
   B   Buprenorphine
   C   Atropine
   D   Diazepam

2. **The dose rate for buprenorphine is 0.006 mg/kg (6 µg/kg). The concentration of the solution is 0.3 mg/ml (300 µg/ml). How many ml does a 50-kg animal require ?**
   A   0.1 ml
   B   0.5 ml
   C   1 ml
   D   2 ml

3. **Which volatile liquid is now rarely used because it is toxic to the myocardium and explosive?**
   A   Chloroform
   B   Trichloroethylene
   C   Cyclopropane
   D   Ether

4. **The Magill circuit is classified as which type of breathing circuit?**
   A   Open
   B   Semi-open
   C   Semi-closed
   D   Closed

5. **Recovery from thiopentone-induced anaesthesia takes place through**
   A   Metabolism of the anaesthetic by the liver
   B   Redistribution of the thiopentone to fatty tissues, and then gradual metabolism by the liver
   C   Excretion of unchanged thiopentone by the kidney
   D   Exhalation of the anaesthetic

6. **All of the following anaesthetics can be used in the dog except**
   A   Ketamine
   B   Propofol
   C   Alphaxalone and alphadolone acetate
   D   Methohexitone sodium

7. **The agent that can be used to reverse the effects of Small Animal Immobilon in man is**
   A   Naloxone
   B   Neostigmine
   C   Atipamezole
   D   Etorphine

8. **Which of the following volatile anaesthetic agents must not be used with soda-lime?**
   A   Isofluorane
   B   Halothane
   C   Chloroform
   D   Trichloroethylene

9. **The pressure in a nitrous oxide cylinder decreases when**
   A   The cylinder is half full
   B   All of the liquid nitrous oxide has vaporized, which occurs only when the tank is nearly empty
   C   The cylinder is heated
   D   The cylinder is initially opened, then the pressure gradually decreases until the tank is empty of pressure

10. **Anticholinergics are often included in premedication for cats and dogs**
    A   To produce pupil dilation
    B   To decrease saliva and bronchial secretions
    C   To decrease the amount of induction agent required
    D   To calm the animal

11. **Which of the following is a narcotic?**
    A   Pethidine
    B   Xylazine
    C   Ketamine
    D   Propofol

12. **Of the following drugs commonly used as premedicants which does not cause a fall in blood pressure?**
    A   Xylazine (Rompun)
    B   Acepromazine
    C   Ketamine
    D   Medetomidine (Domitor)

13. **Soda-lime consists of several compounds. Which chemical compound makes up the majority of the soda-lime?**
    A   Sodium hydroxide
    B   Potassium hydroxide
    C   Calcium hydroxide
    D   Silicates

14. **What capacity is a size E oxygen cylinder?**
    A   680 l
    B   1360 l
    C   3400 l
    D   6800 l

15. **An ataractic is**
    A   A drug which causes drowsiness
    B   A drug which produces calmness without drowsiness
    C   A drug which stimulates respiration
    D   A drug which decreases the sensation of pain

16. **Which of the following is a barbiturate anaesthetic?**
    A   Methohexitone sodium
    B   Alphaxalone and alphadolone
    C   Ketamine
    D   Propofol

17. **A neuro-leptanaesthetic is**
    A   A mixture of an opioid with an analgesic
    B   A mixture of an analgesic with a premedicant
    C   A mixture of a sedative with an inhalation anaesthetic
    D   A mixture of a sedative with an opioid analgesic

18. **MAC numbers have been calculated for all the inhalation anaesthetics. Which of the following has the lowest MAC number?**
    A   Methoxyflurane
    B   Halothane
    C   Nitrous oxide
    D   Isoflurane

19. **Nitrous oxide and oxygen can be used together in anaesthesia. What combination is usually used?**
    A   1:1 Nitrous oxide:Oxygen
    B   2:1 Nitrous oxide:Oxygen
    C   3:1 Nitrous oxide:Oxygen
    D   4:1 Nitrous oxide:Oxygen

20. **The anaesthetic used by Guedel to classify the stages of anaesthesia was**
    A   Chloroform
    B   Halothane
    C   Ether
    D   Thiopentone

21. **Different anaesthetic circuits require different fresh gas flow rates. Which circuit uses 1–1.5 × minute volume?**
    A   Lack
    B   Ayre's T-piece
    C   Bain
    D   Circle system

22. **The dilution of adrenaline usually kept in case of anaesthetic emergencies is**
    A   1 in 10
    B   1 in 100
    C   1 in 1000
    D   1 in 10 000

23. **As an animal becomes anaesthetized, which is the first reflex to be lost?**
    A   Pedal reflex
    B   Anal reflex
    C   Swallowing reflex
    D   Palpebral reflex

24. **According to the Health & Safety Executive, what is the maximum length of tubing suitable for use with a passive scavenging system?**
   A   3 feet
   B   5 feet
   C   8 feet
   D   12 feet

25. **The anaesthetic gas supplied in blue cylinders is**
   A   Oxygen
   B   Nitrous oxide
   C   Carbon dioxide
   D   Cyclopropane

26. **Activated charcoal within a circuit removes which of the following?**
   A   Carbon dioxide
   B   Halothane
   C   Nitrous oxide
   D   Halothane and nitrous oxide

27. **The dose rate for thiopentone is 10 mg/kg, and you have been given a 2.5% solution. How many ml would you need to draw up for a 50-g mouse?**
   A   0.2 ml
   B   0.02 ml
   C   0.5 ml
   D   5 ml

28. **The intravenous anaesthetic with the shortest recovery time is**
   A   Propofol
   B   Thiopentone
   C   Methohexitone
   D   Ketamine with xyiazine

29. **Under Guedel's classification, which stage of anaesthesia is surgical anaesthesia?**
   A   Stage I
   B   Stage II
   C   Stage III
   D   Stage IV

30. Which of the following is a depolarizing neuromuscular blocker?
A Neostigmine
B Suxamethonium
C Naloxone
D Vecuronium

31. Muscle relaxants act at which site within the nervous system?
A The neuromuscular junction
B The nerve axon
C The brain
D The spinal cord

32. The Stephens machine uses which type of anaesthetic circuit?
A Semi-open
B Circle
C To and fro
D Semi-closed

The answers are on page 112

Surgical instruments and equipment

10 Questions

1. **The retractor which is not self-retaining is the**
   A   Langenbek retractor
   B   West's retractor
   C   Gossett retractor
   D   Gelpi retractor

2. **ASIF cortical and cancellous bone screws can be distinguished in which of the following ways?**
   A   Cancellous screws are always fully threaded
   B   Cancellous screws have tighter threads than cortical screws
   C   Cortical screws have a hex screwdriver fitting
   D   Cortical screws are more tightly threaded than cancellous screws

3. **Jacob's chuck is used to apply which orthopaedic implant?**
   A   Plate
   B   Rush pin
   C   Cerclage wire
   D   Intramedullary pin

4. **The needle holders which have scissors combined are**
   A   McPhail's needle holders
   B   Bruce Clarke's needle holders
   C   Olsen–Hegar needle holders
   D   Mayo–Hegar needle holders

5. **The pilot hole for a 3.5 mm ASIF cortical screw should be drilled using which sized drill bit?**
   A   1.5 mm
   B   2.0 mm
   C   2.5 mm
   D   3.5 mm

6. **The forceps which have a rat tooth end are**
   A   Lane's forceps
   B   Bendover forceps
   C   Spey forceps
   D   Allis tissue forceps

7. How should instruments be passed to a surgeon?
   A   Ratchet open, rings first
   B   Ratchet open, tips first
   C   Ratchet closed, rings first
   D   Ratchet closed, tips first

8. Strabismus scissors are used in which particular type of surgery?
   A   Orthopaedic surgery
   B   Aural surgery
   C   Ophthalmic surgery
   D   General surgery

9. The instrument that can be used as a haemostat is
   A   Halsted mosquito forceps
   B   Allis tissue forceps
   C   Adson dissecting forceps
   D   Cheatle forceps

10. Which blade is known as a tenotomy blade?
   A   No. 10
   B   No. 15
   C   No. 11
   D   No. 20

The answers are on page 122

Sterilization and maintenance of an aseptic theatre

10 Questions

1. **In order to move about in the operating room, how should scrubbed personnel pass each other?**
   A   Any way that is convenient
   B   Back to back
   C   Back to front
   D   Front to front

2. **To prepare a skin site for surgery, all of the following procedures are recommended except**
   A   Clip and then prepare the area three times using a surgical scrub solution and then alcohol
   B   Prepare the area centripetally, progressively moving toward the site of the incision
   C   Remove all clipped hair before beginning preparation of the site
   D   Remove all surface dirt before beginning the surgical scrub

3. **Sterilization cannot be achieved by**
   A   Boiling
   B   Autoclaving
   C   Infra-red radiation
   D   Ethylene oxide

4. **If you have scrubbed in order to assist with a surgical operation, in which order should you place the surgical drapes?**
   A   Closest to yourself first, and then proceeding in a clockwise direction
   B   Starting on the opposite side to yourself (the surgeon's side), and then proceeding in a clockwise direction
   C   Starting closest to yourself, then on the opposite side (the surgeon's side), and then the two ends
   D   Any of the above is acceptable

5. **Which statement is not true about hot air ovens?**
   A   Instruments sterilized in this way cannot be packaged
   B   The temperature does not need to be as high as for autoclaves
   C   Sharp instruments need 180 minutes at 150°C
   D   Mineral oil, waxes and petroleum jelly can be sterilized in this way

6. **Theatre design and management should allow for all of the following except**
   A   The minimum number of people should be allowed in theatre at any time
   B   The theatre should have two entrances
   C   The theatre should have an X-ray viewer
   D   Sinks and the scrubbing-up area should not be in the operating theatre, but in a separate preparation area

7. **The holding time for sterilizing instruments for an autoclave operating at a pressure of 15 lb/sq in and a temperature of 121°C is**
   A   3 min
   B   10 min
   C   15 min
   D   30 min

8. **Surgical gloves are sterilized using which sterilization method?**
   A   Infra-red radiation
   B   Gamma radiation
   C   Ethylene oxide
   D   Autoclave

9. **Surgical procedures can be classified according to the degree of asepsis maintained during the operation. Which category would a cystotomy fit into?**
   A   Clean
   B   Clean-contaminated
   C   Contaminated
   D   Dirty

10. **The sterility monitor that responds to temperature and time only is the**
   A   Sterigauge
   B   TST strip
   C   Autoclave tape
   D   Browne's tube

The answers are on page 124

Suture materials and suturing

1. The suture material that remains the longest in a wound before it is broken down by enzymes is
   A   Catgut
   B   Polyglycolic acid (Dexon)
   C   Polyglactin 910 (Vicryl)
   D   Polydioxanone (PDS)

2. Assuming no complications, how long after surgery should skin sutures generally be removed?
   A   2–3 days
   B   4–5 days
   C   7–10 days
   D   15–17 days

3. In old nomenclature, what size suture material is one size thicker than 3/0?
   A   2/0
   B   4/0
   C   1
   D   0

4. Suture patterns are described as being apposing, inverting or everting. Which of the following suture patterns is an everting pattern?
   A   Simple interrupted
   B   Horizontal mattress
   C   Cruciate mattress
   D   Ford interlocking suture

5. Which is the smallest suture material?
   A   0.2 metric
   B   6/0
   C   2 metric
   D   3/0

6. The suture material which is monofilament is
   A   Silk
   B   Catgut
   C   Polypropylene (Prolene)
   D   Polyglactin 910 (Vicryl)

7. **If a curved cutting needle was examined in cross section, how would it appear?**
   A   Triangular with the apex of the triangle on the inside of the curve
   B   Triangular with the apex of the triangle on the outside of the curve
   C   Square, with the corner on the inside of the curve
   D   Round, with a fine, tapered point

8. **How is wire suture material sized?**
   A   Gauge e.g. 20 g
   B   Metric e.g. 6 metric
   C   BPC gauge e.g. 2/0
   D   French gauge e.g. 6 FG

The answers are on page 127

10 Obstetrical and paediatric nursing

Obstetrics and paediatrics

20 Questions

1. **Oestrus can be prevented, suppressed or postponed by using which of the following types of drug?**
   A   Oestrogens
   B   Progestagens
   C   Prostaglandins
   D   Oxytocin

2. **If a lactating bitch was presented at the surgery showing signs of shivering, muscle spasm, collapse and disorientation, which post-parturient condition would you suspect?**
   A   Metritis
   B   Lactation tetani (eclampsia)
   C   Mastitis
   D   Parvovirus

3. **It is essential that neonates receive colostrum within 36 hours of birth or they will not receive the full value of the colostrum. Why is this?**
   A   They cannot digest the proteins
   B   They are unable to absorb the antibodies directly into the blood stream
   C   They lack the enzymes needed to break down the antibodies
   D   The fat content is too high

4. **How long after birth do pups' and kittens' eyes open?**
   A   3–6 days
   B   7–9 days
   C   10–14 days
   D   15–21 days

5. **Which statement about the reproductive cycle of the queen is correct?**
   A   She is seasonally monoestrous
   B   She is non-seasonal
   C   She is a spontaneous ovulator
   D   None of the above

6. **All of the following are types of foetal dystocia except**
   A   Foetal oversize
   B   Breech presentation
   C   Uterine inertia
   D   Foetal monster

7. **The puerperium is the term used to describe**
   A   The period immediately prior to parturition
   B   The period after parturition during which the uterus returns to normal
   C   The foetal membranes that are produced after all the foetuses have been born
   D   The area immediately around the vulva

8. **The hormone present through metoestrus in the bitch is**
   A   Oestrogen
   B   Follicle stimulating hormone
   C   Progesterone
   D   Luteinizing hormone

9. **In the event of a misalliance in the queen, which drug may be given to terminate the pregnancy?**
   A   Oestrodiol benzoate (Mesalin)
   B   Megoestrol acetate (Ovarid)
   C   Proligestone (Covinan)
   D   None of the above

10. **The average duration of oestrus in the bitch is**
    A   4 days
    B   21 days
    C   18 days
    D   9 days

11. A breech birth occurs when a foetus is delivered in

A   Posterior longitudinal presentation, dorsal position, with head and legs extended

B   Anterior longitudinal presentation, ventral position, with head and legs extended

C   Anterior longitudinal presentation, dorsal position, with forelimbs and neck flexed

D   Posterior longitudinal presentation, dorsal position, with hindlimbs flexed

12. If an animal is primigravid it means that

A   She has had a litter before

B   She is only carrying one foetus

C   This is her first litter

D   The uterus is lying in an abnormal position

13. How often would you feed a week-old orphan pup that was being hand reared?

A   Every two hours

B   Every four hours

C   Every six hours

D   None of the above

14. Blood tests can be carried out to determine whether a bitch is ready to be mated or not. Which hormone is tested for?

A   Luteinizing hormone

B   Oestrogen

C   Follicle stimulating hormone

D   Progesterone

15. If a vaginal smear was taken from a bitch during oestrus, which cell type would predominate?

A   Round epithelial cells

B   Red blood cells

C   White blood cells

D   Cornified epithelial cells

16. **What is strabismus?**
    A   Straining to pass faeces
    B   A squint
    C   An inability to crawl
    D   A head tilt

17. **Semen for Artificial Insemination (AI) is usually collected from the tom cat using which of the following methods?**
    A   Electro-ejaculation
    B   Injection of testosterone
    C   Digital manipulation
    D   Artificial vagina

18. **Vaginal smears can be stained using which of the following?**
    A   Leishman's stain
    B   Wright's stain
    C   Difquik
    D   Any of the above

19. **Which of the following species is an induced ovulator?**
    A   Dog
    B   Cow
    C   Ferret
    D   Hamster

20. **At what stage during pregnancy is palpation for pregnancy diagnosis possible?**
    A   1–2 weeks
    B   3–4 weeks
    C   5–6 weeks
    D   Only after 6 weeks

The answers are on page 129

Answers

General nursing

1. A *A decubitus ulcer is a pressure sore*
Decubitus ulcers are common complications in recumbent patients. They occur mainly over bony prominences, where the tissues are deprived of oxygen because the animal's weight compresses the blood vessels supplying the area.

2. C *Higginson's syringe can be used for giving an enema*
Higginson's syringe is a rubber pump that is used to transfer fluid from a container through a bulb that is squeezed and out through a narrow nozzle that is inserted into the animal's rectum.
   Sprawle's needle is a blunt ended metal cannula used for irrigating the ear canal.
   A burette is used in combination with a giving set to deliver a specific volume via a drip. Fluid can be drawn from the thorax or abdomen simply by using a syringe and needle or syringe and catheter. When removing fluid from the thorax it is helpful to use a three-way tap to ensure that air does not enter the pleural cavity. Alternatively a mechanical chest drain can be used with a one-way valve.

3. B *Jackson's catheter should be used for catheterization of a cat*
Jackson's catheter is a short fine urinary catheter with a central wire stylet which helps introduction of the catheter. It has a luer fitting, and a plastic collar with small holes in it, so that it can be sutured to the skin and left as an indwelling catheter.
   Tiemann's, Dowse's and Foley catheters are all used in the bitch.

4. B *If a patient that had undergone oesophageal surgery, a gastrostomy tube would be the most appropriate*
Oesophageal tissues do not heal very easily, and so to avoid trauma to the area food should be given in such a way as to by-pass the oesophagus. The best way is to use a gastrostomy tube. Liquid food can be administered via the tube, and the animal is sure to receive a balanced diet. Animals tolerate gastrostomy tubes well, and they can be placed at the time of surgery, either using an endoscope, or by the use of other commercially available gastrostomy tube applicators.

5. B *You should suggest that they restrict protein in the diet and increase carbohydrate levels*
Protein should be restricted as many older animals start to develop liver and kidney problems. These may not be clinically apparent, but by cutting down on surplus protein, and changing the type of protein to something more readily digestible, it is possible to slow down the rate of deterioration of these organs. The carbohydrate levels require increasing simply to replace the calories that would previously have been supplied by protein.

Water should always be freely available. Acute renal failure can be precipitated by allowing animals to become dehydrated through inadequate fluid intake.

Energy levels should also be monitored closely. Most animals require fewer calories as they get older as their activity levels decrease.

Exercise is important for all animals, including older animals. However, this should be given little and often and on a regular basis to keep joints flexible, maintain the animal's interest and provide ample opportunity for urination and defaecation.

6. B *1 unit French Gauge is 1/3 mm*
Catheters are measured in French Gauge (FG). This gives the external diameter of the catheter.

7. C *A nasogastric tube of diameter 6–8 FG should be used for a medium-sized dog*

8. C *The disease which is not associated with older age is osteochondrosis*
Osteochondrosis is a disease seen in young animals, and usually presents clinically before the animal is a year old.
    Periodontal disease and osteoarthritis are progressive conditions which usually start in middle to old age. Diabetes mellitus is also a disease that is classically seen in the middle-aged animal.

9. B *Dysphagia is difficulty in eating*

10. B *The most serious complication of prolonged recumbency is hypostatic pneumonia*
If an animal is allowed to lie on one side for long periods of time, the lower lung becomes compressed by the animal's weight and is not aerated properly. Bronchial secretions also pool in the lower lung, and this provides an ideal medium in which bacteria can multiply.
    Turning a patient at least every four hours can help prevent this from occurring. Alternatively, propping a recumbent patient in sternal recumbency so that both lungs can be used will help. Coupage of the chest loosens bronchial secretions and enables the ciliated cells lining the respiratory tract to move the secretions up from the lungs.
    Decubitus ulcers, joint stiffness and muscle wastage are all complications of prolonged recumbency, but are generally less life threatening that hypostatic pneumonia. All can be avoided or minimized with good nursing care.

11. C *Constipation in patients can be prevented by the use of high fibre diets*
Fibre helps to prevent constipation by absorbing moisture and keeping the faeces fairly soft and easy for the animal to pass.
    Kaolin is used to treat diarrhoea.

Diagnostic tests

1. A   *A centrifuge would be needed in order to measure packed cell volume (PCV)*
The packed cell volume or PCV is a measurement of the proportion of a blood sample that is made up of cells. This can only be measured by centrifuging the sample so that all the cells are packed closely together with the plasma or serum lying on top.

Haemoglobin estimation either requires colour matching by eye, or the use of a colorimeter. Red blood cell and platelet counts require the use of diluting fluids, a microscope and counting chamber, usually the Improved Neubauer Counting Chamber.

2. B   *The Wintrobe tube can be used for measuring PCV*
The Wintrobe tube was used for measuring PCV before microhaematocrit capillary tubes were available. It is a narrow tube with graduations marked up the side. Blood is introduced into the tube very carefully using a fine pipette to ensure there are no air bubbles. The sample is then centrifuged for 30 minutes at 3000 rpm. The PCV can then be read from the markings on the side of the tube.

3. D   *Dehydration is characterized by increased PCV and increased plasma protein levels*
In dehydration there is a loss of the fluid fraction of blood, so all cells and biochemical parameters are increased. This is true providing there is no pathology other than fluid loss.

4. C   *Variation in erythrocyte size on a blood smear is called anisocytosis*
Spherocytosis means that the cells are not biconcave, but more spherical in shape.

Poikilocytosis means that the cells vary from the normal circular shape.

Anisochromasia means that the cells are not uniformly pigmented, and that there is variation in their colour.

5. D   *When present in urine, ascorbic acid can mask a positive glucose reaction on urine dipsticks*
Dogs are able to synthesize vitamin C (ascorbic acid) in the intestines. If too much is produced it is cleared from the body by the kidney, and so can appear in the urine of normal animals. It affects the tests for glucose as it inhibits the enzymes on the stick tests and produces false negatives, and it increases values for glucose when Clinitest or Benedict's reagent are used, thus leading to false positives with these tests.

6. B   *The specific gravity of urine from this dog is most likely to be between 1.006 and 1.025*
The history and blood results show that the dog is in chronic renal failure. This usually means that the animal is unable to actively concentrate or dilute its urine as the renal tubules are no longer functioning adequately. The concentration of the urine will therefore be the same as the concentration of a filtrate of plasma, usually between 1.010 and 1.012.

7. D   *The most likely haematological abnormality is a decreased platelet count*
An increase in platelet numbers or changes in the PCV would not affect an animal's clotting ability. However, lack of platelets would result in multiple small haemorrhages occurring as minor damage is done to small blood vessels. Normally damage to a blood vessel causes the platelets to change structure slightly and become sticky, so that they clump together and plug the hole. The clotting cascade is then activated, and eventually fibrin is laid down to form a more permanent seal over the site. Without the clotting factors the platelet plug only lasts for about 24 hours and then disintegrates.

8. A *Severe parasitism can result in an eosinophilia*
Parasitic infestations which have systemic effects on the
body stimulate an increase in the numbers of circulating
eosinophils. Eosinophilia is also seen in allergic responses,
and as an ideopathic finding in some individual animals.
There have also been suggestions that increased numbers
of eosinophils are found in animals with rage syndrome.

9. C *The normal PCV for a cat is 24–45%*

10. A *A blood smear for a differential white blood cell count should
be stained using Leishman's stain*
A differential white blood cell count requires the use of a
stain that will allow the identification of all the white
blood cells. In order to do this the dye must have two
components, one dye to highlight alkaline areas, and a
second to show the acidic areas. Romanowsky stains such
as Leishman's stain contain methylene blue, which stains
alkaline areas dark blue, and eosin, which stains acidic
areas red. This enables the white blood cells to be
distinguished and counted.
   Gram's stain is used to distinguish between Gram-
positive and Gram-negative bacteria.
   Lugol's iodine can be used in Gram's stain, or on its
own to locate undigested starch within faecal smears.
   New methylene blue is used as a supravital stain to
identify reticulocytes.

11. C *In a complete blood count, a left shift refers to an abundance
of immature white blood cell forms*
This is most commonly seen in response to bacterial
infection, when many immature neutrophils such as bands
and stabs enter the circulation to counter the infection.
The reason that it is described as a shift to the left is that
if neutrophil development is written as a flow diagram
across the page from left to right, then in this type of
response there are more cells from the left appearing in the
circulation.

12. D *Increased serum amylase and lipase activities usually suggest pancreatic disease*
Inflammation of the pancreas causes release of the digestive enzymes amylase and lipase into the circulation. These are not normally present in the blood stream.

13. A *Urinary casts are produced within the kidney tubules*
These are made of protein that is deposited within the tubules. The tubules act as a mould, and the resulting solid cast contains whatever other substances were present in the tubule at the same time. This can be white blood cells, fats, or epithelial cells from the walls of the tubules. The different appearances of the casts can provide information about pathology within the kidney.

14. B *The test used to detect the presence of protein in urine is the copper sulphate test*
Approximately 1.5 ml of sodium hydroxide is added to the same volume of urine. The same volume of 1% copper sulphate solution is then added. If a purple colour develops, this indicates that protein is present within the urine sample.

Hay's test is used to check for the presence of bile salts. A positive result to Fouchet's test indicates bile pigments, and Benedict's reagent is used to show glucose is present.

15. C *The normal red blood cell count for a dog is $5.5–8.5 \times 10^{12}/l$*
The normal white blood cell count for a dog is $6–18 \times 10^9/l$

16. D *The white blood cells which usually make up 5% of the differential count are monocytes*
Neutrophils account for between 60 and 70% of the white blood cells, lymphocytes between 15 and 20%, and less than 1% of the total white blood cell count are basophils.

17. A *White blood cell diluting fluid contains acetic acid to lyse the red blood cells*

Without the acid, the whole field of view within the counting chamber would be packed with red blood cells which would make the white blood cells hard to identify and count. The diluting fluid also often contains a dye, such as crystal violet or malachite green, to stain the white blood cells and make them easier to see.

18. C *In order to determine a differential white blood cell count, the minimum number of white blood cells that should be counted is 200*

19. A *The enzyme that provides most information about damage to liver cells is ALT*

ALT or alanine amino transferase is an enzyme found within liver cells. In cats and dogs this is the only place it is found, so any increases in serum or plasma levels of this enzyme indicate that there is damage to the liver cells.

AST or aspartate amino transferase is another enzyme also found in liver cells. However, it is not liver specific, and is also found in cardiac and skeletal muscle cells, so damage to any of these cells will result in an increase in blood levels.

Cholesterol is produced by the liver as a by-product of fatty acid metabolism. It can increase in liver disease, but will also increase in other conditions such as hypothyroidism, diabetes mellitus, or if the animal has just eaten.

Bilirubin is a bile pigment, which is normally excreted via the gall bladder into the intestine, and lost from the body in faeces. It is produced as a waste product from haemoglobin breakdown in the circulation, then processed by the liver and made into bile. Increased bilirubin levels can therefore arise in one of three ways: through increased red blood breakdown (haemolysis), liver disease or failure of normal bile excretion into the intestine. An increase in blood levels therefore does not automatically indicate liver disease.

20. A *Alcoholic Sudan III is the stain used to detect undigested fats in faecal smears*
Lugol's iodine is used to detect undigested starch and eosin shows up undigested muscle. New methylene blue is the dye used to identify reticulocytes in blood smears.

21. A *Urate crystals are found in the urine of some Dalmatians as a hereditary condition*

22. D *Urine intended for bacterial studies should be preserved using boric acid*
Universal tubes containing boric acid are usually indicated by having a red cap.
   Toluene is good for preserving urine for chemical examination. Formalin and thymol are good general purpose preservatives, especially for examination of urinary sediments.

23. C *White cell casts in a urine sample collected via catheterization would indicate clinical disease*
White cell casts are only seen in disease conditions such as pyelonephritis or glomerulonephritis. Mucus and spermatozoa are common findings within the urinary tract, and transitional epithelial cells are often seen in urine samples from catheterized patients as the catheterization process displaces them from the walls of the urinary tract.

24. A *When using Leishman's stain, the undiluted stain should be left on the slide for 2 minutes*
It is then diluted using distilled water with pH 6.8, and left for over 10 minutes. The slide is then washed with distilled water and propped up to dry.

25. B *The total magnification of a microscope is calculated by multiplying the eyepiece magnification with the objective magnification*

26. B *The stain used to examine fungi is lactophenol cotton blue*
Gram's stain is used for bacterial identification. Wright's
stain is a Romanowsky stain that can be used for
differential white blood cell counts, and iodine is used
either as part of Gram's stain, or on its own to show
undigested starches within faecal smears.

27. C *A colorimeter measures the amount of light absorbed by a
coloured solution*
Coloured solutions absorb a particular wavelength of light.
The amount of light that passes through the solution is
compared with the light passing through a colourless
solution so that the amount absorbed can be calculated.
    The intensity of the colour of the solution is related to
the concentration of the solution. Therefore if the
absorption for a solution of unknown concentration is
compared with the absorption of a solution of known
concentration, the concentration of the unknown solution
can be determined.

28. B *Before drawing off serum, blood should be allowed to clot for
at least 30 minutes*
However, it should not be allowed to stand for longer
than 2 hours before the serum is removed as the clot starts
to break down after this time.

29. D *The bacterium that needs to be stained using the Ziehl–
Neelsen staining technique is Mycobacterium tuberculosis*
Mycobacterium tuberculosis is one of several bacteria that
are described as being acid fast. They are not stained
easily using Gram's stain or methylene blue, but require
this specialized staining technique.

30. D *A supravital staining technique has to be used to identify reticulocytes*
Supravital staining techniques involve culturing living cells with the stain, so that the dye is taken up into organelles. This technique is used for reticulocytes, immature red blood cells which still contain the remnants of organelles within their cytoplasm. The cells are cultured at 37°C with the dye for 30 minutes immediately after sampling, and then a smear is made in the same way as a blood smear would be made normally.

The dyes that are used in this way are Brilliant Cresyl Blue and New Methylene Blue, and both show the organelles as darker blue strands within the cytoplasm.

31. C *Bilirubin would be found in the urine of a dog suffering from obstructive jaundice*
In obstructive jaundice there is obstruction to the normal outflow of bile from the gall bladder into the small intestine. Therefore bile produced by the liver dams back into the circulation and blood bilirubin levels increase. This is seen clinically as jaundice. Eventually the bilirubin levels exceed the renal threshold and bilirubin is found within the urine.

32. D *The bacteria which would appear as Gram-negative rods under the light microscope are* Escherichia coli
Streptococci and staphylococci are both Gram-positive cocci. The streptococci tend to form chains of organisms, and staphylococci are more likely to be found in clumps.

Clostridia are also Gram-positive, but are short rods.

33. A *The McKenzie brush technique is used as a diagnostic method for ringworm*
Asymptomatic animals are brushed through with a sterile brush, and the brush is then pushed into Sabouraud's medium. The medium is then cultured to see if the animal under assessment is a carrier of the ringworm fungus.

This method is used in multi-animal households or colonies where there have been clinical cases of ringworm, and in-contact animals have to be tested for the infection.

34. C *Cystine crystals are usually hexagonal in appearance*
Struvite (triple phosphate) crystals usually appear like coffin lids. Urates resemble thorn apples, and calcium oxalate crystals are octahedral and are often described as looking like envelopes when viewed through the microscope.

Elementary microbiology

1. C *The difference between Gram-negative and Gram-positive bacteria is that Gram-negative bacteria have an extra cell wall layer*
The extra layer possessed by Gram-negative bacteria is made of lipopolysaccharide (LPS), and is responsible for the different staining characteristics of Gram-negative bacteria compared with Gram-positive bacteria. It also confers some of the pathogenicity of Gram-negative bacteria.

Both Gram-negative and Gram-positive organisms can have flagella, though not all do, and there are pathogenic examples of both types of bacteria.

2. C *Bacteria reproduce by simple binary fission*
Bacteria divide by asexual division, in which the entire contents of a cell are duplicated and then divided equally into two cells. Mitosis is the equivalent type of cell division that takes place in the majority of animal cells.

Conjugation and spore formation are survival techniques used by some bacteria to overcome conditions which are not favourable to their survival. Conjugation occurs in some Gram-negative bacteria and involves the transfer of small pieces of genetic information from one cell to another. Spore formation is seen in some Gram-positive bacteria, and results in the development of a spore which is very resistant to disinfectants, heat and drying. Once conditions improve, the bacterium returns to its vegetative form, and starts to reproduce normally again.

3. C *Structural components of all viruses include a protein capsid and nucleic acid*
Viruses are very simple organisms that only have to consist of a protein shell and their genetic information. The genetic code can be carried as either RNA or DNA. Some viruses are slightly more complex and in addition have other structures such as an envelope, but this is not seen in all types.

4. B *The bacterium which can form spores is* Clostridium tetani
Only certain Gram-positive bacteria can form spores, and
these include the Clostridia and Bacillus species. The
spores can remain dormant for long periods of time within
the environment, until they encounter conditions which are
favourable for growth again.

5. C *Exotoxins are produced by Gram-positive bacteria*
Exotoxins are substances produced and released by some
Gram-positive bacteria. The toxins increase the organism's
virulence or capability to produce disease. They are quite
easily destroyed by heat, but can be very toxic. They are
produced and released while the bacterium is still alive.
    Endotoxins are formed by Gram-negative bacteria.
Endotoxin is the lipopolysaccharide layer of the cell wall,
and so is only released once the bacterium dies.
Endotoxins produce signs of shock when present in large
quantities, but if only a small amount is present then the
signs are of mild fever and malaise. They can withstand
boiling, but are destroyed at temperatures over 120°C.

6. C *Wood's lamp examination will cause some Microsporum
species to fluoresce*
Approximately 60% of Microsporum species will fluoresce
when viewed using an ultra-violet light. The fungus shows
as an apple green fluorescence, usually most obvious at the
edge of a lesion. However, starch and other substances can
produce false positives, and some species do not fluoresce,
so Wood's lamp results should be interpreted with caution.
If the lesion is suspicious, then cultures should be made of
hair plucks from the edge of the area for confirmation of
the diagnosis.

7. B *The type of medium used to culture fungi is Sabouraud's medium*
Selenite broth and desoxycholate citrate agar are both selective media used to encourage the growth of Salmonella bacteria. McConkey agar is another bacterial culture medium used to identify lactose fermenting bacteria that can grown in the presence of bile salts, such as *Escherichia coli.*

8. C *Selenite broth is a selective medium*
Selenite broth is used for the detection of Salmonella bacteria.
  Nutrient agar is a basic agar mix on which most bacteria will grow. Blood agar and chocolate agar contain the same basic nutrients as nutrient agar, but have had blood products added. They are sometimes called enriched media. These types of media are used for some fastidious bacteria which require additional nutrient factors.

9. D *Anaerobic conditions are required to grow Clostridia bacteria*

10. C *An example of a pathogenic yeast is Candida*
Candida is sometimes found in chronic ear infections, and is the organism responsible for sour crop in birds.
  Aspergillus, Trichophyton and Microsporum are all examples of moulds.

11. A *Viruses are measured in nanometres, nm $(1 \times 10^{-9}m)$*
Bacteria are quite a bit larger, these are measured in micrometers, μm $(1 \times 10^{-6}m)$

12. C *The term 'facultative anaerobe' is used to describe a bacterium that can grow in the absence of oxygen, but grows better when oxygen is available*
A bacterium with an absolute requirement for oxygen is an obligatory aerobe.

A bacterium that grows optimally without oxygen is an anaerobe.

A bacterium that grows best in minute quantities of oxygen is a microaerophile.

13. C *Dermatophyte test medium turns red if fungi are cultured on its surface*
Dermatophyte test medium (DTM) is a variant on Sabouraud's medium which contains an indicator which changes colour when a certain sugar is metabolized. Fungi use this sugar preferentially, so the medium changes colour from orange to deep red if they are present. Bacteria can also grow on the medium, but use a different sugar first, and so do not produce the colour change.

Elementary parasitology

1. B *The mite that can cause alopecia around the eyes and muzzle
without obvious pruritus is Demodex canis*
Otodectes cynotis is the ear mite which causes excessive
ear wax production, and intense irritation. Cheyletiella and
Sarcoptes mites both live on the body and produce
pruritus.

2. C *The larval stage of Toxocara canis which is infective is L_2*
When eggs of Toxocara canis are passed in faeces, the
worm starts to develop within the egg. The first and
second stage larvae develop there, and it is when the egg
contains the L_2 larva that it is infective if ingested by an
animal.

3. A *The proper name of the hookworm is Uncinaria stenocephala*
There is also another hookworm occasionally seen in dogs
called Ancylostoma.
   Trichuris vulpis is the whipworm. Oslerus osleri is the
canine lungworm. This used to be called Filaroides osleri.
Toxascaris leonina is an intestinal roundworm similar in
appearance to Toxocara species.

4. B *Linognathus setosus is a sucking louse*
Sucking lice have mouthparts that enable them to suck
blood from their host. Linognathus is the sucking louse of
the dog.
   Trichodectes canis and Felicola subrostratus are both
biting lice which feed off the epidermis. Trichodectes is
found in the dog, and Felicola in the cat. There is no
sucking louse of the cat.
   Ctenocephalides felis is the proper name for the cat flea.

5. A *The larval form of Trombicula autumnalis is parasitic*
The nymph and adult forms of Trombicula are free living,
and it is only the larvae that parasitize cats and dogs. The
mites are often found around the ears or feet, and can
cause marked irritation and self-excoriation.
   Note: Trombicula can also be called Neotrombicula
autumnalis.

6. D *Taenia hydatigena always requires an intermediate host*
Taenia species are tapeworms, and all tapeworms require
an intermediate host as they have indirect life cycles.

Toxocara canis, Toxascaris leonina and Toxoplasma
gondii can all undergo direct life cycles, or may use
another host.

7. D *The parasite which typically causes intense pruritus and
crusting of the ear tips is Sarcoptes scabiei*
This is the way in which many Sarcoptes infestations first
appear clinically, but the mites quickly spread over the
body, and the animal rapidly becomes covered in sores as
it scratches and bites at itself.

Demodex infestations are usually non-pruritic, unless
there is secondary bacterial infection.

Trichodectes and Cheyletiella do cause irritation, but
can be found anywhere over the body.

8. A *Trichuris vulpis has a distinct lemon-shaped egg, with a plug at
each end*
The eggs of Toxascaris and Toxocara are round, and quite
similar to each other, except that the surface of the
Toxocara egg is more pitted.

Uncinaria eggs are oval, and several cells may be seen
within the shell.

9. D *The eggs of Linognathus setosus are glued to the hair shafts of
its host*
All lice produce eggs which they cement to the hairs of the
host. The eggs are often referred to as 'nits'.

10. B *Toxoplasma is not passed from queen to kitten via milk*
Toxoplasma can be transmitted via contaminated food,
sheep abortions or meat from an intermediate host.

11. C *The term which describes infestation by dipteran larvae is myiasis*
Dipteran larvae, or maggots, cause what is usually called fly-strike in animals. Flies lay their eggs on areas of the skin or fur that is soiled with faeces, blood or urine, and when the eggs hatch the maggots start to eat the contaminated tissues, and then continue to burrow their way into healthy tissues.

Mydriasis is the term for pupil dilation and miosis is the opposite, meaning pupil constriction.

Meiosis is the type of cell division seen in the development of the sperm and ova.

12. C *The whipworm of dogs is Trichuris vulpis*
Aelurostrongylus abstrusus is the lungworm of the cat. Oslerus osleri is the lungworm of the dog, and Uncinaria stenocephala is the hookworm.

13. A *Pruritus and excessive epidermal scaling can be caused by the non-burrowing mite Cheyletiella*
Cheyletiella infestations are often seen in young animals, and are often referred to as 'walking dandruff', because of the large amount of epidermal scaling.

Notoedres and Sarcoptes are both burrowing mites, seen in the cat and dog respectively. These also produce significant irritation.

Otodectes cynotis is a non-burrowing mite, but lives solely within the ear canals stimulating increased production of ear wax, and localized irritation.

14. B *Taenia hydatigena reproduces asexually*
All tapeworms are hermaphroditic, that is they contain the sexual organs of both the male and female. Toxocara cati, Ixodes ricinus (the sheep tick) and Felicola subrostratus are all parasites that reproduce sexually.

15. A *Visceral Larva Migrans in man is caused by Toxocara species*
Visceral Larva Migrans occurs when a human is
accidentally infected by Toxocara larvae. Since man is not
the normal host, the larvae undergo part of their life cycle
and migrate through body tissues, before becoming
dormant. In most cases this migration does not produce
significant clinical effects, but in a small number of cases
signs such as liver pain, or neurological signs, are seen.
The occurrence of clinical disease depends on which tissues
the larvae migrate through or where they finish their
migration. In a tiny proportion of cases the larvae lodge in
the retina and provoke a granulomatous reaction which
causes partial or even total blindness in the affected eye.
   Toxoplasma can also affect humans, and is particularly
dangerous for women exposed to the organism for the first
time during pregnancy. In about 10% of cases, this can
lead to damage to the foetus, or even abortion.
   Echinococcus granulosus is another potential zoonosis,
and can produce large hydatid cysts in man in the same
way as it does within its normal intermediate host, the
sheep.

16. D *A paratenic host is a host which carries the immature parasite
within its tissues. It has to be eaten by the final host for the
parasite to complete its life cycle.*
A host in which a parasite has to undergo part of its life
cycle before it can reinfest the final host is an intermediate
host.
   A host which carries an organism and sheds it
intermittently is a transport host.
   An animal in which the adult or reproductive phase of
the parasite's life occurs is called the final or definitive
host.

Infectious diseases

1. D *The cause of feline infectious anaemia is* Haemobartonella felis

Haemobartonella is a rickettsia which attaches itself onto the surface of red blood cells. Affected cells are destroyed as they pass through the spleen and other lymphoid organs, giving rise to anaemia. The organism can be detected by making blood smears and staining them with Giemsa. The organism shows up as purple rings or cocci on the surface of the cells. Several blood samples may need to be taken over a period of time as the organism is not always present within the circulation.

2. C *'Blue eye' is a complication encountered in dogs vaccinated with live canine adenovirus-1 vaccine*

'Blue eye' is so called because the cornea of the eye becomes opaque which gives it a bluish sheen. It is caused by corneal oedema, the result of antigen–antibody complexes lodging within the cornea. It is seen in a very few cases both in the naturally occurring disease, and after vaccination with live attenuated canine adenovirus-1 (CAV-1). In most cases it resolves spontaneously, but in a tiny proportion of cases the pup is left with permanent scarring of the cornea.

To prevent this from occurring, another vaccine is routinely used which contains attenuated canine adenovirus-2 (CAV-2). This provides cross protection for CAV-1, carries no risk of pups developing Blue eye, and also protects against CAV-2, one of the organisms that produces respiratory disease as part of the kennel cough complex.

3. A *The cat should be isolated and retested in two to three months*
Over 40% of cats infected with Feline leukaemia virus (FeLV) recover fully from the virus. These cats mount an immune response against the virus and throw off the infection without the development of FeLV-related diseases. Therefore an apparently healthy cat should be isolated, so that it is no risk to any other cats, and then retested after about 12 weeks. If it is still carrying the virus, then it should be kept isolated and cared for until such time that it develops one of the FeLV-related diseases, and its quality of life deteriorates. If the owner is unable to keep the cat isolated during this period, it is probably best that it is euthanased so that it does not present a risk to other healthy cats in the area.

4. B *The incubation period for parvovirus in dogs is 3–5 days*
Most viruses have quite short incubation periods. Leptospira bacteria have a longer incubation period of between 7 and 21 days, and kennel cough has an incubation period of between 5 and 10 days.

5. C *Feline herpes virus 1 can become latent after an initial infection*
After a primary infection, cats infected with feline herpes virus apparently recover. However, the organism remains latent, or hidden, within the body where it is held in check by the immune system. If the cat is stressed in some way, then the herpes virus is able to multiply within tissues, and clinical signs redevelop. The main sign seen with herpes virus infection in cats is upper respiratory tract disease.

6. D *Leptospira organisms may be found in both the blood and urine of infected animals*
Animals with leptospirosis undergo bacteraemias in which the bacteria circulate within the blood stream, and eventually settle in either the liver or kidney or both, depending on the particular organism. They often remain within the interstitial tissues of the kidney for many months after the clinical signs of the disease regress, so urine from clinically recovered animals can still contain viable bacteria. This is important with regards to disease control.

7. B *Chlamydia infection in a cat can be diagnosed by microscopy of conjunctival scrapings*
The scrapings are stained with Giemsa, and intracytoplasmic inclusion bodies can be seen in affected cells.

8. B *A fomite is an inanimate object that becomes contaminated by a pathogenic organism and then comes into contact with a non-infected animal*
Organisms which are not easily destroyed once out of the host are often passed in this way.

9. C *The fleas act as transport hosts for* Haemobartonella felis
Transport hosts are animals which carry a particular organism unchanged and are able to shed the organism at any time.
Biological vectors are hosts which are required by an organism for it to undergo part of its life cycle. Immature forms of the organism are found in the biological vector, and they are then passed on to a final host where the adult or reproductive phase of the organism's life cycle occurs. Intermediate hosts are the same thing, except that the term intermediate host is reserved for biological vectors which carry the immature stages of parasites.

10. C *Canine adenovirus-1 can cause acute pyrexia, petechial haemorrhages on the gums, hepatic enlargement, possible neurological signs, collapse and death in affected dogs*
Canine adenovirus-1 (CAV-1) causes the disease canine infectious hepatitis.

Acute myocarditis or gastro-enteritis is seen in parvovirus infections.

Canine distemper virus produces several different clinical syndromes including respiratory signs, hyperkeratosis and neurological signs.

The group of organisms which form the kennel cough complex give rise to respiratory signs.

11. D *Leptospirosis is zoonotic*
Canine parvovirus, distemper virus and canine adenovirus-1 are all host specific, and will not affect humans.

12. B *A saprophyte is an organism that lives on dead organic matter*
An organism that lives on a larger organism and causes disease is described as being pathogenic. Organisms that benefit their hosts are symbiotic or mutualistic, and organisms that do not have any effect on their hosts are described as commensals. However, if the immune system of the host is compromised, many commensals can become opportunist pathogens.

13. C *Viral diseases can be positively diagnosed in the live animal by checking for a rising antibody titre*
Paired blood samples are taken from the animal approximately two weeks apart, and antibody levels to the particular organism are measured. Animals which show an increase in the antibody levels are actively mounting an immune response against the infection, and therefore are definitely carrying the virus.

14. C *The organism responsible for Feline infectious peritonitis is not resistant to many disinfectants, and does not remain in the environment for very long*
Feline infectious peritonitis (FIP) is caused by a coronavirus. The virus is readily destroyed by most disinfectants, and is easily killed by heat and drying. However, its mode of transmission is not well understood, even apparently isolated households can be affected by the disease and the incubation period is very variable. Two forms of FIP are seen clinically: the wet form, in which a proteinaceous fluid forms within body cavities, and the dry form, in which micro-abscesses develop in the major organs of the body.

15. C *Canine parvovirus is thought to have evolved from feline panleucopaenia virus*
Feline panleucopaenia (also called Feline infectious enteritis) is caused by a parvovirus which results in severe enteritis. The canine parvovirus is very similar, so similar in fact, that when canine parvovirus infections were first seen, feline enteritis vaccines were used in dogs to minimize the spread of the disease.

16. C *Feline calici virus causes chronic stomatitis and gingivitis*
Feline calici virus is one of the feline viruses which can cause chronic infections in cats. Affected animals may continue to shed the virus throughout their life, and often redevelop clinical signs. Chlamydia psittaci can also do this, though the signs associated with this organism tend to be ocular discharges and conjunctivitis.

17. A *Canine parvovirus can last in the environment for up to a year*
The parvoviruses are very resistant to many disinfectants, heat and desiccation, and therefore can remain viable within the environment for long periods of time.

18. B *Isolated cases should always be treated after the remainder of the in-patients*

Potentially infectious or contaminated animals should always be handled and treated last, so that the risk of disease transmission from these animals to those without infections is minimized. Ideally, infectious patients should be looked after by someone different from the person dealing with the rest of the animals, but this is not always possible. Protective clothing should always be worn, and nursing staff should disinfect themselves going into and out of an isolation ward. Isolation areas should have their own sets of food bowls, bedding and cleaning materials, so that nothing has to come out of the isolation area.

19. D *A neonate exposed to the Feline leukaemia virus is most likely to become persistently infected with the virus*

Cats exposed to Feline leukaemia virus (FeLV) before the immune system has had a chance to develop have the highest chance of becoming persistently infected, and eventually suffering from the FeLV-related diseases. Cats over four months of age have a much better survival rate after exposure. Up to 40% of these animals will recover from infection without long-term problems.

Kittens born from vaccinated cats, which have received maternal antibodies via colostrum, are less at risk than those born of unvaccinated queens.

Immunity and vaccination

1. C *Cellular immunity involves the activities of monocytes and T-cells*

T-cells are one of two different types of lymphocyte. When an antigen enters the body it is picked up by circulating monocytes which present it to different T-cells. Eventually a T-cell is encountered that responds specifically to the particular antigen. This stimulates the proliferation of the T-cell into several different types of T-cells which can all respond to the antigen. This type of immunity is described either as cellular immunity or cell-mediated immunity. It does not involve the production of antibodies.

2. C *Mature antibody-producing cells are called B-cells*

These are the second type of lymphocyte. Like the T-cells, they are specific for a particular antigen. Monocytes pick up the antigen and present it to B-cells until a correct match is found. This causes the B-cell to multiply and start producing antibodies against the antigen.

3. B *Animals are not routinely vaccinated before they reach eight to nine weeks of age because there may still be maternal antibodies within the plasma*

After an animal is born, it receives maternal antibodies from colostrum, which enter the neonate's blood stream. These antibodies can last within the circulation for up to 16 weeks, but numbers gradually decline after about four to six weeks. If a vaccine is given while there are still high levels of circulating maternal antibodies the young animal has no need to produce its own antibodies, as the maternal antibodies act against the antigen. However, after the maternal antibodies have broken down, there is no residual immunity. If the vaccine is given once maternal antibody levels have decreased, then the immune system of the pup or kitten is stimulated to produce its own response, which has a much longer lasting effect.

4. C *A toxoid contains antigen from a toxin*
A toxoid is something that mimics a toxin without causing the tissue damage a toxin would produce. It stimulates an immune response to the toxin.

Antigen from a micro-organism is used within vaccines to stimulate an immune response to the organism.

Antitoxin contains antibodies to a particular toxin, and antiserum, sometimes called hyperimmune serum, contains antibodies to an organism. These do not stimulate an immune response, but simply provide immediate protection for an animal. They are usually used in the face of disease.

5. D *The canine infectious disease which is always protected against using a dead vaccine is leptospirosis*
Parvovirus, distemper and infectious canine hepatitis can be protected against with the use of either live or dead vaccines.

6. B *Dead vaccines are less long lasting in effect that live vaccines*
Dead vaccines do not multiply within the animal so they only produce a relatively limited immune response. They require at least two injections for the initial vaccination course, and regular boosters to maintain the level of protection.

They are very safe since the organism is dead, so cannot produce disease. However, because the immunity produced is not as good as for live vaccines they are less widely used now than the live types.

7. B *Live attenuated vaccines should be stored between + 2 and + 8°C*

8. A *The release of interferon is stimulated by infection with a virus*
Interferon is released by virus-infected cells. It acts on
neighbouring cells and protects them from infection by the
virus. It is not specific to one particular virus; the same
reaction will take place whatever the type of virus.

This does not occur after infection with any other
organism.

Medical diseases and their nursing

1. D *Diets containing restricted levels of protein and sodium should be given to animals with renal failure*

Protein should be restricted to avoid the build up of toxic metabolites such as urea, which cannot be cleared quickly from the body by the diseased kidneys. Sodium should also be restricted to prevent fluid retention and the development of hypertension.

High fibre diets can be used in the management of animals with colitis. Food allergies should be treated using very simple diets which contain nutrient sources that the animal has not encountered before.

Cats with feline urologic syndrome (FUS) require diets which have restricted mineral contents, and which result in the production of urine which has a pH that does not encourage the development of uroliths.

2. A *A hyperthyroid cat would not show bradycardia*

Hyperthyroid animals produce excessive amounts of the thyroid hormones T_3 and T_4. These hormones drive the animal's metabolism, and in excess result in very high metabolic rates. The clinical signs of weight loss, polyphagia, heat intolerance, mild diarrhoea and tachycardia are the result of the metabolic changes.

3. D *The cardiac disease which is congenital is persistent right aortic arch*

Persistent right aortic arch arises because the aorta develops from the right aortic arch rather than the left in the embryo. As a result, the oesophagus becomes trapped between the aorta, the ligamentum arteriosum and the pulmonary vein. The circulatory system functions perfectly normally, but clinical signs are seen as food does not pass through the narrowed oesophagus easily, and so the animal starts to regurgitate food and a megaoesophagus develops cranial to the stricture. The ligamentum arteriosum can be transected surgically, but it may be too late for the oesophagus to return to normal in which case the animal will need to be fed semi-liquid food from a height, so that gravity helps it slide down into the stomach.

Endocardiosis is seen mainly in older animals. Nodules develop on the valvular flaps and prevent them from closing properly. The condition worsens gradually and may eventually lead to the development of heart failure.

Cardiomyopathies can arise either as primary conditions, or secondary to other diseases such as hyperthyroidism in cats. The heart muscle is affected so that it no longer functions adequately to maintain cardiac output.

Myocarditis is inflammation of the cardiac muscle. This usually develops as the result of some type of infection, for example parvovirus in very young pups. It is quite rare.

4. A *The clinical sign not typically associated with small intestinal diarrhoea is tenesmus*

Tenesmus, or straining, is most commonly seen with large intestinal problems.

In small intestinal diarrhoea weight loss is common since the animal is not able to digest or absorb its food normally, and as a result of this it is usually ravenously hungry. Borborygmi or increased gut sounds are also common.

5. D *Keto-acidosis can develop as a complication of diabetes mellitus*

In diabetes mellitus there is an absence of insulin needed to drive glucose into cells. The cells therefore have to use an alternative energy source, and will use fatty acids and glycerol instead. Metabolism of these molecules leads to the formation of acidic ketone compounds as by-products. These accumulate within the circulation and can lead to life-threatening acidosis.

6. C *An animal suffering from left-sided heart failure would show pulmonary oedema leading to a cough*

In left-sided heart failure, the left ventricle is not able to push sufficient blood into the systemic circulation to meet the body's demands. A 'back-log' of blood develops in the left atrium, and dams back into the pulmonary circulation.

As pressure in the pulmonary vessels increases, fluid is pushed out of the capillaries into the alveolar spaces, and pulmonary oedema develops.

In right-sided failure a similar situation arises, except that the blood accumulates within the systemic circulation, so that the major veins become distended and central venous pressure increases. This can cause a jugular pulse, and ascites and oedema to develop. The heart muscle hypertrophies in response to cardiac failure. The right side enlarges in right-sided failure, and the left increases in left-sided failure.

7. A *Furunculosis is a severe example of pyoderma*
Furunculosis is a very deep skin infection, often caused by anaerobic bacteria. The most common sites for it to develop are around the anus, especially in German Shepherds with low tail carriage, and in the feet.

8. C *The insulin with the longest duration of action is Insuvet protamine zinc*
Insuvet protamine zinc lasts for about 36 hours, and has peak activity after 12–24 hours.

Insuvet neutral is a soluble insulin that can be given by intravenous injection. This has a very rapid onset of activity, but only lasts for about two hours.

Insuvet lente is a medium-acting insulin with peak activity after 6–12 hours, and total duration of 24 hours.

Caninsulin is a mixed insulin and has peak activity after 3–12 hours, and an active life-span of 8–24 hours.

9. C *Salt should be decreased in patients with cardiac disease*
Reducing salt levels decreases water retention by the body, and therefore helps to lower blood pressure. Reducing the circulating blood volume decreases the workload on the heart, and prevents rapid deterioration of the patient's condition.

10. D *Jaundice can be caused by either increased red blood cell destruction, bile duct obstruction or liver disease*
Jaundice develops when there is excess bilirubin within the circulation. Bilirubin is produced as a waste product of haemoglobin breakdown, and is normally processed by the liver and excreted via bile into the intestine.

If any of these processes are affected by disease, then there can be an increase in blood bilirubin levels resulting in jaundice.

11. D *Arterial blood pressure is at its maximum during ventricular systole*
The term systole is used to describe cardiac muscle contraction, and diastole describes relaxation of the muscle. The period during which arterial pressure is at its maximum is when the ventricles are actively contracting and pushing the blood into the arteries, which is ventricular systole.

12. D *Hepatic encephalopathy is seen in cases of chronic liver disease due to the toxic effects of amino acids and ammonia within the blood stream*
The initial breakdown products of protein metabolism are amino acids and ammonia. The ammonia is toxic to the central nervous system, and is normally deaminated and converted into slightly less toxic products such as urea by the liver. In liver failure this does not take place, and if the animal continues to eat a high protein diet, the ammonia levels increase, leading to neurological signs.

High levels of urea will develop if the kidneys are damaged, and this will also cause neurological signs if left untreated.

Chronic liver disease does result in lack of the plasma proteins, as these are normally synthesized by the liver. However, this leads to the development of ascites and oedema, not neurological signs.

13. B *The bone condition associated with chronic renal failure is Rubber jaw (secondary hyperparathyroidism)*
In renal failure phosphate is retained within the circulation. The calcium–phosphorus balance is therefore upset, and parathyroid hormone (PTH) is released to increase blood calcium levels to restore the balance again. PTH stimulates bone resorption, so that eventually they become weakened and soft. This is particularly noticeable in the jaw. If the mandibles of anaesthetized patients with this condition are squeezed gently, there is abnormal bending of the bones. This is painful if tried in the conscious animal.

Marie's disease is a condition in which there is bone proliferation on the distal long bones, causing pain and lameness. This occurs in response to the presence of intrathoracic masses, although it is not well understood why.

Lion jaw is another proliferative bone disease. The mandibles of affected animals are inflamed, and it is painful for the animal to open and close its mouth. There may be new bone laid down around the temporo-mandibular joint which restricts the range of movement of the joint. It is most commonly seen in West Highland White Terriers. The cause is not understood, but in most cases progression of the disease stops once the animal reaches skeletal maturity.

Barlow's disease or metaphyseal osteopathy is another disease with no clear cause. The metaphyses (the areas adjacent to the growth plates) are enlarged, and are hot and painful for the animal. Damage can extend to the growth plate and cause limb deformities, but in most cases the condition resolves completely as the animal gets older.

14. B *Foods allergies can be diagnosed using restriction diets*
Animals with suspect food allergies should initially be kept on very simple diets containing foods that they have not encountered before. If the allergy signs improve, then new foods can be added, one at a time, until the symptoms return and the problem food identified.

Intradermal testing can be used to identify contact or inhaled allergens.

Antihistamines will mask the clinical effects of allergies, regardless of the cause, and so are of no use in diagnosis, although they are widely used in the treatment of allergies and atopies.

15. D *The hormones responsible for calcium regulation are parathyroid hormone and calcitonin*
The thyroid hormones control metabolic rate.

Glucocorticoids are released in response to stress to keep blood glucose levels high. Mineralocorticoids are needed to maintain sodium and potassium balance within the body.

Insulin and glucagon are responsible for the regulation of blood glucose levels.

16. B *Pentobarbitone can be used in the management of a fitting animal*
In cases of status epilepticus pentobarbitone (Sagatal) is often used to induce a long-lasting anaesthesia. The brain's activity is suppressed, and the hope is that once the effects of the anaesthetic wear off, the focus of the epileptic fit will remain quiet.

Phenyl propanolamine (Propalin) is used in the treatment of urinary incontinence.

Prednisolone is a short-acting glucocorticoid that can be used to treat inflammatory or auto-immune conditions.

Phenylbutazone is a non-steroidal anti-inflammatory widely used in the management of osteoarthritis.

17. D *The hormone released by the kidney when blood pressure falls is renin*

Renin is released as soon as glomerular perfusion decreases. It stimulates the conversion of inactive angiotensinogen in the circulation, into the active form, angiotensin. Angiotensin causes vasoconstriction, and so increases blood pressure, and also stimulates the adrenal cortex to release the hormone aldosterone. Aldosterone encourages sodium retention, so that water is also retained, and blood pressure is further increased.

Erythropoietin is also produced by the kidney, but is produced continuously. It acts on the bone marrow to stimulate the maturation of red blood cells.

18. C *Endocardiosis causes the development of nodules on the cusps of the heart valves, which prevents them opening and closing normally, and is the most common cause of congestive heart failure in the dog*

This is common, especially in certain breeds, such as the Cavalier King Charles Spaniel. Clinical signs start to show as the animal reaches middle age, and worsen with age.

Pericardial effusions result from several different conditions, including infections or tumours. Fluid accumulates within the pericardial cavity, causing compression of the heart, especially the weaker right side. The heart can no longer pump efficiently and signs of heart failure develop.

Endocarditis is the result of blood-borne infections reaching the endothelium of the heart, causing inflammation and disease. Animals are normally pyrexic and lethargic. Long courses of systemic antibiotics are needed to treat these cases.

Myocarditis is inflammation of heart muscle, again usually caused by infection. This is quite rare now, although it used to be seen in very young pups with acute parvovirus infections.

Poisons

1. A *The specific antidote which can be given to an animal suspected of having been poisoned with lead is sodium calcium edetate in saline solution*
Ethanol and sodium bicarbonate are used for ethylene glycol poisonings. Atropine sulphate is the antidote for organophosphorus toxicity, and acetyl cysteine can be given after paracetamol poisoning.

2. C *Animals with ethylene glycol poisoning often develop calcium oxalate crystals within their urine*

3. D *Chronic lead poisoning leads to the development of nervous signs*
The signs seen include disorientation, ataxia and blindness.
   Many poisons produce vomiting and diarrhoea as clinical signs, so these should not be regarded as diagnostic for any particular poison.
   Acute interstitial pneumonia is seen after poisoning with paraquat.
   Changes in coat pigmentation are not usually seen in small animal poisoning cases.

4. D *The pesticide with an anaesthetic action, which causes a dramatic drop in body temperature and leads to hypothermia and death, is alphachloralose*
This is found in some rodenticides.
   Sodium chlorate affects haemoglobin within the blood, and causes depression, anorexia, abdominal pain and haematuria.
   Paraquat is a very potent poison, leading to depression, vomiting, diarrhoea, progressive dyspnoea and death within ten days.
   Metaldehyde produces neurological signs including incoordination, loss of consciousness, convulsions and cyanosis.

5. D *Acetyl cysteine can be used in the management of animals suspected of having been poisoned by paracetamol*

6. D *Vomiting should not be induced if poisoning by bleach, phenol or petroleum products is suspected*

Vomiting should not be induced in any patient that is unconscious, convulsing or that has ingested an irritant or volatile poison. Bleach and phenol are both very irritant, and petroleum products are volatile.

7. C *Warfarin is used legally as a rodenticide*

8. D *Carbon monoxide, sodium chlorate and paracetamol all produce changes in haemoglobin which lead to a colour change of the blood*

Sodium chlorate and paracetamol both change haemoglobin into methaemoglobin. This results in the mucous membranes appearing a muddy brown colour.

Carbon monoxide is carried by haemoglobin in preference to oxygen, and instead of the blood appearing a dark red colour, it lightens to a cherry red colour. This can be misleading, because without looking carefully, the animal can appear to have a healthy colour suggesting that normal oxygenation of tissues is occurring. In fact, the tissues are hypoxic as carbon monoxide cannot be used by the tissues and there is little oxygen available.

Fluid therapy

1. B *The dog requires 1000 ml for rehydration*
If the dog is 8% dehydrated, it has lost 8% of its body weight.
   Calculate 8% of the body weight $= 8/100 \times 12.5$ kg
                                       $= 1$ kg
This is the weight of the fluid that has been lost.
   But 1 litre of water weighs 1 kg, therefore this dog has lost 1 litre of fluid.
   1 litre $= 1000$ ml, therefore the fluid deficit for this dog is 1000 ml.

2. D *The fluid that should be used intravenously to maintain an animal once it is rehydrated is 0.18% sodium chloride, 4% dextrose (1/5 normal saline)*

3. B *The drip should be set to provide 1 drop every 2 seconds*
You need to give 2160 ml in 24 hours.
   Therefore you need to give
                    2160/24 ml in 1 hour
             $= 90$ ml/hour
             $= 90/60$ ml/min
             $= 1.5$ ml/min
   But 1 ml $= 20$ drops, therefore
             $= 1.5 \times 20$ drops/min
             $= 30$ drops/min
             $= 30/60$ drops/sec
             $= 0.5$ drops/sec, or 1 drop every 2 seconds

4. A *Sodium bicarbonate should not be given with Hartmann's solution*
Hartmann's solution contains calcium ions. If sodium bicarbonate was added to Hartmann's solution it would react with the calcium to produce solid calcium carbonate which would precipitate out within the drip. Ringer's solution also contains calcium ions, so sodium bicarbonate should not be used with this either.
   Sodium bicarbonate is used in cases of severe acidosis to absorb excess hydrogen ions within the body, and can be given with normal saline, 5% dextrose or 0.18% sodium chloride in 4% dextrose.

5. B *Over-infusion of intravenous fluids could lead to the development of oedema*

If over-infusion of intravenous fluid occurs the circulation becomes overloaded, and blood pressure increases. This forces fluid out of capillaries into the interstitial spaces. This is evident as oedema. The site of oedema development depends on the type of fluid being infused. Colloids remain in the circulation, which increases the workload of the heart. Eventually the heart is unable to cope and blood dams back into the pulmonary circulation leading to pulmonary oedema.

Crystalloids do not remain in the circulation, but equilibrate throughout all the fluid compartments. Therefore the whole body becomes saturated with fluid, and oedema forms in all tissues.

6. C *Plasma forms approximately 5% of an animal's total body weight*

The total fluid within the body accounts for between 60 and 70% of an animal's body weight. This is divided into intracellular fluid (40–50% of body weight) and extracellular fluid (20% of body weight). The ECF is divided further into the interstitial fluid (15% of body weight), plasma and lymph (5% of body weight), and the transcellular fluids (<1% of body weight).

7. A *Unconsciousness results in a primary water deficit*

A primary water deficit occurs when there is loss of fluid from the body without electrolyte losses. This can arise in any situation where either the animal is unable to drink, or where insensible losses through respiration and sweat are increased. Possible causes therefore include water deprivation, unconsciousness and heat stroke.

Vomiting, diarrhoea and burns all result in dehydration, with the loss of electrolytes as well as water.

8. A *The anticoagulant which is used when collecting blood for blood transfusions is acid citrate dextrose*
Heparin is the anticoagulant used for biochemical studies. EDTA is used for haematology, and fluoride oxalate prevents clotting in samples for glucose assessment.

9. A *Normal central venous pressure in small animals is 3–7 cm water*
Central venous pressure can be measured using a jugular catheter attached to a giving set, a three way tap and a water manometer.
Arterial pressure is far higher than venous pressure, and is measured in millimetres of mercury (mmHg). Normal arterial pressures for cats and dogs are about 150–160 mmHg.

10. D *1.8% sodium chloride is not isotonic*
Almost all the crystalloid fluids routinely used in veterinary practice are isotonic. This means that they exert the same osmotic pressure as fluid within cells, so that giving these intravenously does not cause water to move into or out of the cells through osmosis.

11. C *Hartmann's fluid would be the most suitable to use to rehydrate an animal with chronic diarrhoea*
An animal suffering from chronic diarrhoea would have lost a considerable amount of water, and also would have lost many electrolytes from the intestinal secretions. The most important of these would be sodium and bicarbonate. Hartmann's fluid contains sodium, calcium and lactate. It does not contain bicarbonate because the calcium would precipitate out as calcium carbonate. However, the lactate is metabolized into bicarbonate within the body.

12. D *The cat requires 280 ml of fluid*
For every 1% increase in packed cell volume (PCV) the
animal has lost 10 ml/kg

Therefore, calculate the increase in PCV

$$= 44 - 37 \qquad = 7\%$$

Then calculate the deficit per kg

$$= 7 \times 10 \text{ ml/kg} \qquad = 70 \text{ ml/kg}$$

Then calculate the total deficit

$$= 70 \times 4 \qquad = 280 \text{ ml}$$

13. A *Potassium might need to be supplemented in the drip of an
anorexic cat being maintained on intravenous fluids*
Animals which are not eating, or which have been starved,
will be deficient in many electrolytes including sodium and
potassium. The hormone aldosterone produced by the
adrenal cortex is responsible for maintaining sodium levels
within the body and is released if sodium concentrations
fall. It acts on the renal tubules to conserve sodium and to
excrete potassium ions in exchange.

However, potassium is essential for normal fluid balance
within the body and for normal nerve and muscle
function, and without it cardiac dysrhythmias and muscle
weakness can develop. Animals which are being given
prolonged fluid therapy should therefore be given
additional potassium.

Radiography

1. D *The grid factor for a grid depends on the grid ratio, the lines per inch and the thickness of the lines*
The grid factor is the number by which the mAs has to be multiplied when using the grid to give the same radiographic density as if the grid was not present.

2. B *Scattered radiation is produced due to the Compton effect*
When an incident X-ray of high energy hits an electron, some of the energy of the X-ray photon is given to the electron which is knocked out of position. The X-ray photon continues as scattered radiation, but now has less energy than originally, and may now travel in a completely different direction to that of the primary beam.

The photoelectric effect also occurs as the result of an X-ray interacting with an electron, but occurs with lower energy X-rays. In this case, all the energy of the X-ray photon is transferred to the electron which it displaces. If the displaced electron occupied a position close to the centre of the atom, then an electron from a more distant site can fall into the space now created. As it does so, a tiny amount of radiation, called the characteristic radiation, is released. This is absorbed by the patient.

3. B *The new exposure factors are FFD = 70 cm, kV = 45 kV, mA = 15 mA*
In every calculation regarding exposure factors the mAs should be calculated first. This gives an indication of the number of X-rays reaching the film.

$$mAs = 20 \times 0.3 = 6 \text{ mAs}$$

If the time or the mA have to be changed, the mAs should always remain the same to maintain the same radiographic density.

Therefore New mA × New time = 6 mAs

New mA × 0.4 = 6 mAs

To determine the New mA, divide both sides by 0.4

New mA = 6/0.4 = 15 mA

4. C *The radiation-sensitive grains are found in the emulsion layer of the X-ray film*
The supercoat is a protective layer that overlies the emulsion.

   The subbing layer sticks the emulsion to the polyester base which provides the support for the emulsion.

5. D *Altering the kV will affect the quality of the X-ray beam*
The quality of the X-ray beam is related to the energy of the X-ray photons within the beam. This is controlled by changing the kV which alters the potential difference between the cathode and the anode. If the difference between the cathode and anode is increased, the electrons will travel faster across the vacuum, and the X-rays produced will have higher energy.

   The mA controls the current through the wire filament which results in the release of the electrons. Increasing the current means more electrons are available to move across the tube head, and so more X-rays will be produced. Similarly, increasing the time means that the potential difference is applied for longer, and more electrons have time to cross from the cathode to the anode, so more X-rays will be produced.

   Changing the focal–film distance alters the density of the final radiograph. If the distance is increased, then the energy of the X-rays reaching the plate is the same, and the number of X-rays is the same, but they are spread over a wider area.

6. D *The absorption of X-rays by a tissue depends on its atomic number, the density and the thickness of the tissue.*
The absorption of X-rays depends on all three factors. Therefore bone, which is very dense, and iodine, which has a high atomic number, are radiopaque and show up white on radiographs. Conversely, gas, which has a relatively low atomic number and is not dense, is easily penetrated by X-rays and shows up black on radiographs.

7. D *Unexposed silver bromide grains are washed off the film in the fixer*
During processing, the developer converts exposed silver bromide grains into black metallic silver. The fixer removes any unexposed silver bromide to leave the final image.

8. C *Low osmolar, non-ionic water-soluble iodine preparations should be used as contrast media for myelograms*
These materials are the most inert of all the contrast media, and therefore produce the least damage to the central nervous system, and the least side-effects.
The high osmolar water-soluble iodine-containing compounds can be used for intravascular contrast studies, and for examination of the upper urinary tract, since they are excreted by the kidneys.
Barium compounds are usually used for gastro-intestinal contrast studies, either given orally or per rectum.

9. B *The maximum dose of radiation that a member of the public may legally receive to the whole body is 5 mSv*
The maximum permissible doses (MPDs) are arbitrary doses thought not to carry a significant health risk. Members of the public, including veterinary nurses, should receive less than these doses in a year. Designated workers, such as those dealing with larger radiation sources, have a different set of MPDs. The figures given are for adults over 18. People under 16 should receive no dose at all, and those between the ages of 16 and 18 have intermediate MPDs.

10. D *The use of X-rays in practice is controlled by the Ionizing Radiation Regulations 1985*
The Ionizing Radiation Regulations 1985 is a very complex piece of legislation, so Guidance Notes for the Protection of Persons against Ionizing Radiations arising from Veterinary Use were drawn up. This is not a piece of legislation, but an explanation of the law as it applies to veterinary practices.

11. B *A film that had been overexposed would have a black background, and the subject would also be too dark*
Overexposure means that either too many X-rays have reached the plate, or that the X-rays had too much energy and so were able to pass through the subject too easily. The exposure factors should be reduced to correct this fault.

A film in which the background is black, but the subject is white, has been underexposed. In most cases this means that the X-rays lacked sufficient energy to pass through the tissues, and the kV should be increased to rectify this.

If a film has a grey background, and it is possible to see a finger held up behind it, then it is suggestive of underdevelopment. This could be that the film was not developed for long enough, or that the developer chemical was becoming exhausted, or that the temperature of the developer was too cold.

Finally, if one area of the radiograph was black, it could be because the film had been exposed to light in some way. The box of film could have been left open, or the cassette might not have been closed properly.

12. C *If the distance between the effective focal spot and the film is trebled, then the mAs should be increased by 9 times to maintain the same radiographic density*
As the focal–film distance is increased, the area over which the X-rays are spread becomes greater. The Inverse Square Law states this mathematically:

'The intensity of the X-ray beam is inversely proportional to the focal–film distance squared.'

To compensate for the decrease in intensity the mAs has to be increased. If the distance is trebled, the mAs has to be increased by a factor of 3 squared, i.e. 9.

13. D *X-rays are not reflected by any materials*
They are not reflected, but are able to penetrate all materials to some degree. X-rays travel in straight lines, and will cause blackening of photographic emulsion.

14. B *Parallel grids can result in grid cut-off at the edge of the radiograph*

The primary beam is not a parallel beam, but diverges towards the edge of the area being radiographed. Angled X-ray photons at the edge are unable to pass between the vertical slats of a parallel grid, and so fewer X-rays reach the plate. This phenomenon is called grid cut-off.

Pseudo-focused and focused grids are designed to compensate for this. However, these grids are not identical. Focused grids have slats that are progressively sloped at the same angle as the X-rays within the primary beam, so that they are vertical in the centre, but become more angled towards the edge of the grid. Pseudo-focused grids have vertical lead slats that get shorter and shorter towards the edge of the grid, so that the angled X-ray photons can pass between them and reach the plate.

The Potter–Bucky grid is a moving grid. It moves very rapidly backwards and forwards during the exposure so that grid lines are not visible on the final radiograph.

Regardless of the type of grid being used the exposure factors have to be increased since some of the primary beam X-rays are absorbed as well as scattered X-rays.

15. C *Heat is lost by radiation through the vacuum in the rotating anode X-ray tube head*

In the stationary anode tube head, heat is lost from the target by conduction through a copper rod to the oil bath. This method cannot be used in the rotating anode tube head, because it would conduct the heat to the motor and damage it. Radiation is therefore the only means by which the heat can be lost.

Convection and evaporation are impossible as there is no medium within the tube head, just a vacuum.

16. A *The rectifier within the X-ray tube head is needed to convert*
alternating current into direct current
A step-down transformer changes the mains voltage to
10 V, and a step-up transformer is present to produce the
kilovoltages needed between the cathode and anode of the
tube head.

There is also an autotransformer within the tube head
which smooths out fluctuations in the mains voltage, so
that radiographic quality is consistent.

17. C *Non-screen film should be left in the developer 1 minute longer*
than for screen film, if being processed manually at 20°C

18. C *The settings kV = 80 kV, mA = 40 mA, time = 0.2 sec,*
FFD = 70 cm could be used
First calculate the original mAs

$$\text{Original mAs} = 20 \times 0.2 = 4 \text{ mAs}$$

Then introduce the grid factor 4 to give the new mAs

$$\text{New mAs} = 4 \times 4 = 16 \text{ mAs}$$

Then check the answers you have been given to see if
any of them give an mAs of 16, without changing any of
the exposure factors other than the time and the mA.

In this example there are no answers that fit.

There is, however, a rule of thumb that can be applied if
the mAs becomes too high. Increasing the kV by 10 means
that the mAs can be halved, and this will result in
radiographs of the same appearance.

Therefore, if the kV is increased to 80 kV, the mAs can
be reduced to 8 mAs.

Now check the possible answers for one with these
factors.

19. B *The radius of the controlled area from the X-ray tube head*
when used in an unconfined area is 2 m

20. C *The average lead apron decreases the primary beam by three-quarters*

This still means that a quarter of the primary beam can pass through protective lead clothing, and this presents a significant hazard to the operator. Lead clothing is, however, much more effective against scattered radiation, reducing this to one-twentieth of its original strength. Therefore, lead aprons and gloves should never be considered sufficient protection against the primary beam, only against the possibility of scattered radiation reaching an operator.

21. C *Grids cannot be used to decrease the production of scattered radiation*

In fact, grids result in more scatter being produced, because the exposure factors have to be increased to compensate for their use. What the grids do is to prevent the final image being disrupted by the effects of scattered radiation reaching the film.

Compressing the part being radiographed decreases the thickness of the tissue, and so will cut down the scatter produced. However, this technique is not often used as it could compromise or harm the patient in some way or it is impossible because the tissue being radiographed is bony.

Collimating tightly reduces scatter by limiting the radiation to just the amount needed to produce a diagnostic film. The use of lead-backed cassettes helps by reducing backscatter.

22. B *The use of screens does not mean that higher exposure factors are required than without screens*
Screens contain crystals of materials, such as calcium tungstate, that fluoresce when exposed to radiation. X-ray film is both light sensitive and radiation sensitive, so this means that a single X-ray photon passing through the screens and film will cause both a direct effect on the film and an indirect effect due to the light from the fluorescent crystals within the screens. The screens therefore amplify the effect of the radiation, and so reduce the number of X-rays needed.
   The light produced by the crystals spreads for a short distance in all directions, so that the use of screens does decrease the definition of the radiograph slightly.

23. B *The aluminium filter in the window of the X-ray tube head absorbs any low energy X-rays*
When X-rays are produced, most have the same energy, but there are also some with lower energies. These would be too weak to be of any diagnostic value, but would still contribute to the biological hazard to the patient and operators, so these are removed by an aluminium filter which is placed over the window through which the primary beam passes.

24. C *Developer solutions should be kept in a tank with the lid on to prevent oxidation of the chemicals*
As the chemicals are oxidized they become exhausted, so by keeping the lid on, the useful life-span of a solution is increased.

General surgical nursing

1. D *Paracentesis is not a laparotomy approach*
Paracentesis is the removal of fluid from the abdomen via a needle or catheter.

The pararectal approach describes an incision made parallel but to one side of the midline, parallel to the rectus abdominis muscle.

The paracostal approach is made parallel to the costal arch, following the line of the last rib.

The sublumbar or flank approach is the laparotomy approach most frequently used for cat speys.

2. D *The Ehmer sling can be used after luxation and replacement of the hip joint*
If the shoulder joint is dislocated, then a Velpeau sling can be used after its replacement.

Robert-Jones bandages could be used if support was needed after treatment of stifle or elbow dislocations.

3. C *Shock does not cause a marked parasympathetic response*
Shock is a condition in which there is progressive deterioration of the circulation, so that there is decreased delivery of oxygen to the tissues. It is an emergency situation, since without treatment the vital organs become so hypoxic that they are unable to function adequately, and death follows. Shock can be caused by anything that seriously affects the circulation. Shock can be categorized into three types:

1. Hypovolaemic shock, caused by blood loss or dehydration
2. Maldistributive shock, caused by severe vasodilation which results in a fall in blood pressure and failure of tissue perfusion
3. Cardiogenic shock, caused by heart failure. This is rare in small animals.

4. C   *A gastropexy might be indicated in the management of a gastric torsion*

In a gastric torsion, the stomach twists about the oesophagus which prevents the stomach contents from exiting normally into the intestine. The gastric secretions continue to be produced, and the stomach becomes progressively enlarged with fluid and gas. This causes compression of the vena cava which compromises venous return to the heart. The blood supply to the stomach wall is also affected, since the vessels are trapped in the twist. Without rapid treatment animals with gastric torsions will die, and even those that do receive treatment may die later due to the effect of toxins released into the blood stream when the stomach is returned to its normal position.

To prevent a torsion recurring a gastropexy can be performed, in which the stomach is sutured to the body wall to fix it in position.

5. A   *A wedge biopsy would provide the most information about a lump that was suspected of being a tumour*

If a small 'pie slice' of a lump is taken, fixed in formalin solution, and sent for histopathology, thin slices can be prepared for examination. Since the sample submitted contains cells from the edge and the centre of the lesion the sample should be truly representative of the whole lesion. An accurate diagnosis should then be possible.

A needle biopsy can be used in situations where it is not possible to remove the whole lump. However, the sample taken is much smaller than a wedge biopsy, and there is a chance that the cells collected may not be typical of the cell types present.

Needle aspirates are less accurate still, as literally only a few cells are collected and squirted out onto a slide so that a smear can be made. This technique is most often used in the diagnosis of lymphosarcoma, where the presence of abnormal lymphocytes can be diagnostic.

Exfoliative cytology is really only of use in situations where none of the other techniques are feasible. In this method cells are collected from the surface of the lump. For nasal or prostatic examinations a solution of sterile saline is flushed back and forth over the area, and then collected. It is then spun down and the sediment examined. It is quite common to get non-diagnostic samples using this method.

6. C *Intra-ocular pressure is not decreased in glaucoma*
In glaucoma there is an increase in intra-ocular pressure due to lack of drainage of the aqueous humour in the anterior compartment of the eye. It can be caused either by trauma or through an inherited condition. Left untreated the pressure within the globe increases to the degree that the retina is damaged, and the animal starts to lose vision in the affected eye.

7. D *The Yorkshire Terrier shows an increased incidence of tracheal collapse*

8. C *Urethral calculi could be an indication for performing a urethrostomy in a male animal*
Urethral calculi can often lodge in the narrow urethra of the male animal. In the cat it usually occurs in the terminal urethra close to the penis. In the dog the calculi often lodge at the base of the os penis. It may be possible to flush the calculi back into the bladder when this occurs, but if it is a recurrent condition, it may be better to create a permanent urethrostomy above the point at which the calculi lodge. Diet modifications should also be made to try and prevent the formation of the calculi.

Ruptured bladder, ectopic ureters and hydronephrosis all require surgical management. Hydronephrosis usually requires a nephrectomy of the affected kidney and removal of the ureter. Ectopic ureters can be implanted into the trigone of the bladder, and a ruptured bladder should be surgically repaired.

9. A *Histamine and prostaglandins are natural inflammatory mediators*

Histamine and prostaglandins are released by mast cells and damaged cells after tissue injury. They stimulate capillary dilation and increase capillary permeability. They also attract white blood cells to the area.

10. B *A transverse fracture of a long bone could be repaired using a plate*

A transverse fracture of a long bone is an unstable fracture. There would tend to be rotation of the fragments relative to each other unless they were fixed in some way. Casts, intramedullary pins and splints would prevent most types of movement at the fracture site, but would do nothing to provide rotational stability. A bone plate is the only repair device that could provide sufficient immobilization of the fracture fragments to allow the bone to heal.

11. A *Animals with lymphosarcoma are most commonly treated using chemotherapy*

Several cytotoxic drugs have been used in the management of lymphosarcoma. These include vincristine (Oncovin), cyclophosphamide (Endoxana) and prednisolone. It is important during treatment that the patient's red and white blood cell counts are monitored, since the drugs are toxic to all dividing cells, not just cancerous cells, and bone marrow suppression is a potential side-effect.

Surgery, and complete excision of tumours, is the management of choice for single growths, but is not always possible. Radiotherapy can be used for some tumours that are difficult to operate on. These need to be reasonably superficial, such as oral or nasal tumours, to achieve adequate penetration of the tumour by the radiation. Radioactive isotopes are used only rarely since the patients need to be hospitalized somewhere with adequate radiation protection facilities. Isotopes are sometimes used in the management of thyroid tumours using radioactive iodine.

12. C *Fracture disease is the term used to describe weakening of a bone when a repair device takes all the strain*
Bones are living tissue, and respond to the stresses and strains placed upon them. If a fracture repair device can support the animal's weight, then the bone itself does not need to regain its strength, and may in fact weaken with time. This is fracture disease, and healing will not take place.

Osteomyelitis is infection of the bone.

Malunion occurs when the bone heals, but the alignment is abnormal.

When implants such as plates and screws are being used, it is essential that they are made of the same metal. If they are not, an electric current is set up between them, and the bone becomes damaged by electrolysis. Eventually the implants loosen and fall out, and bone healing will not occur.

13. C *The first thing that should be tried when dealing with a suspect gastric torsion is to pass a stomach tube*
If passing a stomach tube is successful, it will allow gas and fluid to be released from the stomach. This will decrease the pressure on the vena cava and on the gastric wall, and slow the development of severe shock. It is a non-invasive technique that could save the animal's life.

If this does not work, then the next thing to do would be to trocharize the abdomen using a large gauge needle. This should only be carried out under a vet's direction. This also reduces the pressure on the vena cava and provides more time to prepare for other procedures such as surgery.

14. C *An osteochondroma is a benign tumour*
Tumours which have names ending in -sarcoma or -carcinoma are malignant tumours. The only exception to this is the malignant melanoma, which should strictly be called a melanocarcinoma. Most melanomas in small animals are malignant.

15. D *Temperatures as low as −150°C can be reached using liquid nitrogen for cryotherapy*

This is the temperature that can be reached using liquid nitrogen with a probe. Using the liquid nitrogen as a spray even lower temperatures, down to −196°C, can be achieved.

Gaseous nitrous oxide can also be used as a cryogen, but temperatures only reach −50°C with this.

16. B *The lens is affected in the development of cataracts*

Cataracts are opacities that develop on or within the lens. Some cataracts can be removed to leave the lens intact, others can only be treated by surgical removal of the lens (lentectomy).

17. D *Gangrene is the death of tissues with or without bacterial invasion*

18. A *If an animal is suffering from keratitis, the cornea is inflamed*

Inflammation of the conjunctiva is called conjunctivitis, and blepharitis is the term used when the eyelids are inflamed. If the sclera becomes inflamed, then it is described as scleritis or episcleritis.

19. B *Rush pins are often used in pairs in the repair of epiphyseal fractures*

Rush pins are small bone pins with a hook at one end, and a sledge runner tip at the other. They are placed obliquely so that the sledge runner tip contacts, but does not pass through, the opposite cortex of the bone. They are useful for epiphyseal fractures as they cause minimum disruption to the growth plate and the bone can continue to grow as well as heal.

The Steinmann pin is the large intramedullary pin frequently used in orthopaedic surgery. This would not be suitable for the repair of this type of fracture as it is unlikely that the pin would have sufficient hold on the small epiphyseal fragment.

The Kuntscher nail is another type of intramedullary pin. It has either a V- or clover-shaped cross section which gives a better hold than the Steinmann pin within the medullary cavity.

20. B *A drain could be used for a deep wound in which dead space has been created by the surgical removal of some tissue*
A drain is a device that allows air to enter and fluid to flow from deep tissues to the surface. They are often used after tissue removal to allow serum to drain from the area and prevent it accumulating in the dead space.

Anaesthesia and analgesia

1. B *The premedication agent which has significant analgesic effects is buprenorphine*
Buprenorphine is an opiate that produces good analgesia and some central nervous system depression.

Acepromazine produces mental calmness at low doses, but is a sedative at higher doses. Atropine is used for its effects in countering the production of saliva in the anaesthetized patient.

Diazepam is a tranquillizer. It is particularly useful in older patients as it produces minimal respiratory or cardio-vascular depression.

2. C *A 50-kg animal will require 1 ml*
First calculate the dose needed

$$= \text{Dose rate} \times \text{body weight}$$
$$= 0.006 \times 50 \text{ mg}$$
$$= 0.3 \text{ mg}$$

Then calculate the volume needed
$$= \text{Dose/concentration}$$
$$= 0.3/0.3 \text{ ml}$$
$$= 1 \text{ ml}$$

3. D *Ether is rarely used now, since it is toxic to the myocardium and explosive*
Cyclopropane is also explosive, but is not a volatile liquid at atmospheric pressure. It is supplied in pressurized cylinders so that the gas is in liquid form.

Chloroform is a volatile liquid and was used quite extensively in the past, but it causes damage to the patient's liver and kidney, particularly in small animals.

Trichloroethylene is a volatile liquid but it is not widely used as it stimulates respiration, making the depth of anaesthesia hard to monitor.

4. C *The Magill is classified as a semi-closed circuit*
There are four categories of anaesthetic circuits.

The open circuit consists of nothing more than an anaesthetic-soaked gauze held up to the patient's nose. This is sometimes referred to as the 'rag and bottle' method.

The semi-open circuit is a similar arrangement with a gauze pad soaked in anaesthetic, except that there is a head collar or other device that prevents the animal from breathing around the pad.

The semi-closed method includes the majority of anaesthetic circuits such as the Magill, T-piece, Lack and Bain. The patient is given a controlled gas supply which contains a specific amount of anaesthetic agent, and exhaled gases are vented away from the animal.

A closed circuit is one in which the patient rebreathes exhaled gases after the removal of carbon dioxide. This is usually achieved through the use of a soda-lime canister. Examples of this type of circuit include the To and fro circuit, or the Circle system.

5. B *Recovery from thiopentone-induced anaesthesia takes place through initial redistribution of the thiopentone to fatty tissues, and then gradual metabolism by the liver*
Thiopentone is very lipid soluble, and after affecting the brain to produce anaesthesia, is redistributed through all the fatty tissues of the body. The concentration in the brain falls so the animal wakes up. However, there is still thiopentone within the body tissues, and this is then metabolized and removed by the liver over a much longer period of time.

Thin animals have little body fat, so the thiopentone remains within the central nervous system tissue for longer, and recovery is prolonged.

6. C *Alphaxalone and alphadolone acetate must not be given to dogs*

This mixture, marketed as Saffan, must not be used in dogs as they can develop anaphylactic reactions to the 20% cremophor solution which is the carrier for the steroids.

Ketamine can be used in dogs, but only in combination with other drugs such as xylazine (Rompun) or medetomidine (Domitor).

Propofol (Rapinovet) and methohexitone sodium (Brietal) can be used safely in dogs as anaesthetic agents.

7. A *The agent that can be used to reverse the effects of Small animal immobilon in man is naloxone (Narcan)*

Small animal immobilon contains two components: etorphine, an opiate, and methotrimeprazine, a sedative. Naloxone (Narcan) reverses the opiate part of the combination, but the sedative effects persist. Immobilon is an extremely dangerous drug, and should only be used in the presence of someone who is able to give the antidote in case of accidental self-administration.

Neostigmine is used to reverse the effects of non-depolarizing neuromuscular blocking agents.

Atipamezole (Antizedan) is the antidote to the sedative medetomidine (Domitor).

8. D *Trichloroethylene must not be used with soda-lime*

If trichloroethylene and soda-lime are mixed, several noxious products are produced, including phosgene and hydrochloric acid. Trichloroethylene is usually coloured with a blue dye to prevent this occurring accidentally.

9. B *The pressure in a nitrous oxide tank decreases only when all of the liquid nitrous oxide has vaporized, and the tank is almost empty*
Pressure gauges on cylinders which contain gases in a liquid form cannot be used as a means of estimating the quantity of agent remaining. The pressure gauge only indicates the pressure of the gas above the liquid. This stays constant until there is no liquid remaining. The only way to tell how much gas is left is to weigh the cylinder and compare it with the weights of full and empty cylinders. The empty cylinder weight or tare is stamped on the side of the cylinder valve block.

10. B *Anticholinergics are often included in premedication for cats and dogs to decrease saliva and bronchial secretions*
The anticholinergics antagonize the effects of the parasympathetic nervous system, and decrease the unwanted autonomic effects produced by these neurones. The anticholinergics also have other effects which are not necessarily beneficial, such as increasing heart rate, and producing pupil dilation. The most commonly used drug of this type is atropine sulphate.

11. A *Pethidine is a narcotic*
The term narcotic is used to describe drugs that are derived from opium. Narcotics include pethidine, morphine, buprenorphine, butorphanol and codeine.
   Xylazine (Rompun) and medetomidine (Domitor) are both examples of α_2-agonists which produce marked sedation.
   Ketamine is a cyclohexanone, and is sometimes described as a dissociative anaesthetic because of the effect it produces in man.
   Propofol is a water-insoluble phenol which produces both rapid induction and recovery from anaesthesia.

12. C *Ketamine does not produce a fall in blood pressure*
Ketamine causes an increase in heart rate, so that blood
pressure remains normal, or may even be increased.
Ketamine also causes increased muscle tone and muscle
twitching, and should not be used in the dog on its own.

Xylazine and medetomidine produce a transient increase
in blood pressure before causing a marked hypotension.
Acepromazine also produces hypotension, especially when
high dose rates are used.

13. A *Sodium hydroxide makes up the majority of soda-lime*
Soda-lime consists mainly of sodium hydroxide, with
about 10% calcium hydroxide, some silicates and pH
indicators. The sodium hydroxide and calcium hydroxide
react with carbon dioxide and water from the exhaled gas
to remove the carbon dioxide and produce calcium
carbonate. The pH indicators change colour as the soda-
lime is used, and provide an indication of how much of
the soda-lime is left unchanged.

Silicates are included within soda-lime to reduce the
formation of an irritant dust.

14. A *A size E oxygen cylinder contains 680 l*

15. B *An ataractic is a drug which produces calmness without
drowsiness*
The benzodiazepines and acepromazine (used at low dose
rates) are examples of ataractics.

Drugs which cause drowsiness are sedatives.

Analeptics are drugs which stimulate the central nervous
system, and include doxapram (Dopram) which is used to
stimulate the respiratory centre within the brain.

Drugs which decrease the sensation of pain are
analgesics.

16. A *Methohexitone sodium is an example of a barbiturate anaesthetic*
Methohexitone sodium (Brietal) is a barbiturate that is more rapidly metabolized by the liver than thiopentone, and so is more suitable for use in lean animals.
   Alphaxalone and alphadolone (Saffan) are steroids. Ketamine is a cyclohexanone, and propofol is a phenol.

17. D *A neuro-leptanaesthetic is a mixture of a sedative with an opioid analgesic*
Neuro-leptanaesthetics are drug combinations which can be used in a variety of species. Small and Large animal immobilon and hypnorm are examples of drugs used for this type of anaesthesia. They produced marked respiratory and cardiovascular depression, and poor muscle relaxation. Often the animals still remain sensitive to external stimuli such as sound.

18. A *Methoxyflurane has the lowest MAC number*
MAC is an abbreviation for minimum alveolar concentration, and MAC numbers are used as a means of describing the potency of a particular anaesthetic. The minimum alveolar concentration is a measurement of the concentration within the alveoli that is needed to prevent a response to a particular stimulus. The concentration is expressed as a percentage. Anaesthetics with low MAC numbers are therefore more potent than those with high numbers.
   Methoxyflurane has a MAC number of 0.23, halothane 0.8, nitrous oxide 188 to 220 and isoflurane 1.3.
   Nitrous oxide has a MAC number of over 100 because it is impossible to give sufficient agent on its own to prevent a response to the particular stimulus. It only has weak anaesthetic and analgesic properties. However, it is useful in combination with other anaesthetic agents.

19. B *The combination usually used is 2:1 Nitrous oxide:Oxygen*
Nitrous oxide is often used with oxygen as a carrier gas in
inhalation anaesthesia. It has weak anaesthetic and
analgesic properties, which means that the dose of
anaesthetic agent required can be reduced.

It is very readily taken up by haemoglobin within blood
cells, even more so than oxygen, so it should never exceed
80% of the gas mixture or hypoxia could arise. At the end
of anaesthesia the nitrous oxide should be turned off and
pure oxygen administered for at least three minutes. This
is to allow the nitrous oxide to be exhaled before the
animal starts to breathe air, which only contains about
20% oxygen.

Nitrous oxide should not be used if there is a gas-filled
area within the animal's body such as a gastric dilation or
pneumothorax. Nitrous oxide readily diffuses into these
areas, and compromises the animal by increasing the
pressure within the tissue.

20. C *The anaesthetic used by Guedel to classify the stages of
anaesthesia was ether*
Most of Guedel's observations are still true for the modern
anaesthetics, although stages I and II, the induction stages,
are passed through quickly and are not very obvious with
intravenous agents.

21. A *The Lack circuit requires the use of 1–1.5 × minute volume*
To prevent the patient rebreathing, semi-closed anaesthetic
circuits require a minimum fresh gas flow rate. The Lack
and Magill need 1–1.5 × minute volume (the amount of
air an animal breathes in and out in one minute). The
Ayre's T-piece and the Bain use higher fresh gas flow
rates, 2.5–3 × minute volume.

The minute volume is often estimated as 200 ml/kg,
though this will vary considerably for individual animals
depending on age and disease conditions, respiratory rate
and the procedure for which the animal is being
anaesthetized.

22. C *The dilution of adrenaline usually kept in case of anaesthetic emergencies is 1 in 1000*

23. C *As an animal becomes anaesthetized, the first reflex to be lost is the swallowing reflex*
The swallowing reflex is lost quite early in anaesthesia. Once it has been lost, the airway is usually protected by the use of endotracheal tubes with inflatable cuffs which prevent any secretions or vomit entering the trachea while the animal is unconscious. Endotracheal tubes should only be removed once the swallowing reflex has returned.
    The pedal reflex, anal reflex and palpebral reflexes can all be used during anaesthesia to determine whether the patient is under light, medium or deep surgical anaesthesia.

24. C *According to the Health & Safety Executive, the maximum length of tubing suitable for use with a passive scavenging system is 8 feet*
Passive scavenging relies on the gas flow from the anaesthetic machine, and the patient exhaling to drive the contaminated gas through the ducting and out of the theatre. If the tubing is too long, then the gases will pool within the piping, and re-enter the operating theatre once surgery finishes. It also means that the resistance against which the patient has to breathe is quite high.

25. B *The anaesthetic gas supplied in blue cylinders is nitrous oxide*
All the anaesthetic gases are supplied in colour-coded cylinders. Oxygen comes in black cylinders with a white neck. Carbon dioxide is supplied in grey cylinders, and cyclopropane is found in orange cylinders.

26. B *Activated charcoal within a circuit removes halothane*
In some passive scavenging systems adsorbers containing activated charcoal are used. These only remove halothane. If nitrous oxide is being used, this still constitutes a potential hazard for the operators.
    Soda-lime removes carbon dioxide, but does not affect either nitrous oxide or halothane concentrations.

27. B *You would need to draw up 0.02 ml of thiopentone for the mouse*

This calculation needs to be carried out in three stages.

First calculate the dose of agent needed by the mouse
$$= \text{Dose rate} \times \text{body weight}$$

Convert the mouse weight into kg
$$= 50/1000 \text{ kg}$$
$$= 0.05 \text{ kg}$$

$$\text{Dose needed} = 10 \times 0.05$$
$$= 0.5 \text{ mg}$$

Secondly, convert the concentration of the thiopentone from % into mg/ml
$$2.5\% = 2.5 \text{ g in } 100 \text{ ml}$$
$$= 2.5 \times 1000 \text{ mg in } 100 \text{ ml}$$
$$= 2500 \text{ mg in } 100 \text{ ml}$$
$$= 25 \text{ mg in } 1 \text{ ml}$$
$$= 25 \text{ mg/ml}$$

Finally, calculate the volume needed
$$= \text{Dose/concentration}$$
$$= 0.5/25 \text{ ml}$$
$$= 0.02 \text{ ml}$$

28. A *The intravenous anaesthetic with the shortest recovery time is propofol*

If propofol (Rapinovet) is given as a single bolus, it is very rapidly metabolized by the liver, and the animal recovers quickly.

Methohexitone sodium is also broken down by the liver fairly rapidly.

29. C *Under Guedel's classification, surgical anaesthesia is Stage III*
Guedel used ether on human patients to classify the stages
of anaesthesia.
Stage I is the stage of voluntary excitement.
Stage II is the stage of involuntary excitement. Stages I
and II are passed through during induction of anaesthesia.
Stage III is surgical anaesthesia and is divided into 3
planes: plane 1 is light, plane 2 is medium and plane 3 is
deep anaesthesia.
Stage IV is the stage of overdosage.

30. B *Suxamethonium is a depolarizing neuromuscular blocker*
Neuromuscular blockers or muscle relaxants prevent
nervous impulses reaching skeletal muscles and produce
paralysis. There are two types of blocker: depolarizing
blockers, such as suxamethonium, and non-depolarizing
blockers, such as vecuronium, gallamine, atracuronium
and pancuronium.
Non-depolarizing drugs are reversed by neostigmine.
There is no true antidote for the depolarizing blockers, but
neostigmine partially reverses their effects. Neostigmine
should always be used with an anticholinergic such as
atropine.

31. A *Muscle relaxants act at the neuromuscular junction*

32. B *The Stephens machine uses a circle system*
This anaesthetic machine incorporates a closed circle
circuit which contains valves so that gases only flow in one
direction. There are two soda-lime canisters which remove
the exhaled carbon dioxide from within the circuit.

Surgical instruments and equipment

1. A *The retractor which is not self-retaining is the Langenbek retractor*

The Langenbek retractor is a hand-held retractor, whereas the West's, Gossett and Gelpi retractors are all self-retaining.

2. D *Cortical screws are more tightly threaded than cancellous screws*

Cortical screws are designed for use in dense cortical bone. The shaft is wider than the shaft of cancellous screws of the same diameter, and the thread is tighter. Cortical screws are usually fully threaded.

Cancellous screws can be fully or partly threaded, and are designed for use in the loose cancellous or woven bone found in the heads of long bones. These have more widely spaced threads than the cortical screws and narrower shafts.

Both cortical and cancellous screws have a hex screwdriver fitting.

3. D *Jacob's chuck is used to apply intramedullary pins*

4. C *The needle holders which have scissors combined are the Olsen–Hegar needle holders*

5. C *The pilot hole for a 3.5 mm ASIF cortical screw should be drilled using a 2.5 mm drill bit*

The quoted diameter of a screw is diameter of the widest part of the thread. If a 3.5 mm hole was drilled, a 3.5 mm screw would simply drop through without biting.

6. A *The forceps which have a rat tooth end are Lane's forceps*
Lane's forceps are one of the most commonly used tissue forceps.

Spey forceps and Bendover forceps are atraumatic dressing forceps with plain ends.

Allis tissue forceps are self-retaining forceps with a ratchet used for retracting tissue. They have small serrations on the jaws to help grip, but are not as severe as the rat tooth end.

7. C *Instruments should be passed to a surgeon with the ratchet closed, rings first*

8. C *Strabismus scissors are used for ophthalmic surgery*
These are small, delicate scissors used for fine surgery of the eye.

9. A *Halsted mosquito forceps are used as a haemostat*
Allis tissue forceps are used for holding tissues out of the surgical field.

Adson dissecting forceps are a type of rat tooth forceps used for general surgery.

Cheatle forceps are used to transfer sterile items from one place to another by a non-sterile person.

10. C *The No. 11 blade is known as a tenotomy blade*
This is a fine pointed blade which can be used for splitting tendons.

Sterilization and maintenance of an aseptic theatre

1. B *Scrubbed personnel should pass each other back to back*
Passing back to back minimizes the risk of contaminating the most important sterile area, the front of the person. However, it is also important that a scrubbed person does not turn their back on the operating table.

2. B *The area should not be prepared centripetally working in towards the site of the incision*
When a surgical site is prepared, the scrub solution should always be applied working outwards from the site of the skin incision, and never back towards the centre.
   Before starting the surgical scrub it is always important to ensure that as much gross contamination and hair has been removed from the site as possible.

3. A *Sterilization cannot be achieved by boiling*
Boiling will produce disinfection, but not sterilization, as it will not kill bacterial spores. Autoclaving, infra-red radiation and ethylene oxide can all be used to sterilize equipment.

4. C *Drapes should be placed closest to the person placing the drapes first, then the opposite side and then the two ends*
The drape closest is placed first so that the sterile person placing the drapes does not risk contamination by leaning across and touching the patient. The drape on the opposite side can then be placed, so that the surgeon or second scrubbed person can come close to the patient safely. Finally the two end drapes are placed and all are held in place with towel clips.

5. B   *Hot air ovens do not require lower temperatures than autoclaves*
Operating temperatures for hot air ovens are between 150°C and 180°C depending on the substance being sterilized. The temperatures for autoclaves lie between 121°C and 134°C depending on the pressure generated.

Instruments being sterilized by hot air oven are laid out on perforated trays ready for use. The hot air should be able to circulate freely around the instruments, therefore the oven should not be overloaded. Sharp instruments start to blunt with repeated heating, and so should be sterilized using the coolest temperature, 150°C, for 180 minutes. Since no moisture is used in this technique petroleum jelly, powders and other chemicals can be sterilized by hot air ovens.

6. B   *An operating theatre should not have two entrances*
A theatre should only have one entrance, so that it is not a thoroughfare to any other room, and only the minimum number of people are present during an operating session. The theatre should be for surgical procedures only, with all preparation of the patient, surgeon and assistants carried out in a separate preparation area.

It is very helpful for there to be X-ray viewing facilities in theatre.

7. C   *The holding time for sterilizing instruments in an autoclave operating at a pressure of 15 lb/sq in and a temperature of 121°C is 15 minutes*

8. B   *Gamma radiation is used to sterilize surgical gloves*
Gamma radiation is used for most disposables including surgical gloves, suture materials, catheters and needles. Infra-red radiation is used for syringes.

9. B *A cystotomy would be classified as a clean-contaminated operation*
A clean operation is one in which there is no break in asepsis, and none of the uro-genital, respiratory or gastro-intestinal tracts are entered.

A clean-contaminated operation is one in which a contaminated area is entered, but there is no spillage of the contents. This constitutes a minor break in asepsis.

A contaminated operation is when there a leakage from the gastro-intestinal or uro-genital tracts or marked inflammation. There is, however, no infection present. Contaminated surgery includes the management of open, fresh traumatic wounds.

A dirty operation is one in which there is pus and infection present.

10. D *The sterility monitor that responds to temperature and time only is the Browne's tube*
Browne's tubes can be used in either an autoclave or hot air oven, providing the correct tube is chosen. After the specified temperature and time are reached the liquid inside the tube changes from red to green.

Sterigauge and TST strips respond to temperature, steam and time, and so are useful for monitoring autoclave efficiency.

Autoclave tape only shows that steam has penetrated the area where the tape was positioned. It does not give any indication that the correct temperature was reached, or that the steam was present for the appropriate amount of time. This is the least reliable method of testing for sterility.

Suture materials and suturing

1. D *The suture material that remains the longest within a wound before it is broken down by enzymes is polydioxanone (PDS)*
Polydioxanone loses half its strength in 50 days, but is not totally absorbed until after 180 days. Polyglactin 910 (Vicryl) and polyglycolic acid (Dexon) are totally absorbed after about 100 days. Catgut is the suture material which lasts the shortest time. Plain catgut is totally broken down in 15 days, whereas chromic catgut, which is more commonly used, lasts for 30 days.

The way in which absorbable suture materials are removed from wounds depends from what they are made. Natural suture materials, such as catgut, are removed by phagocytosis, whereas synthetic sutures are removed by enzymes which cause hydrolysis.

2. C *Assuming no complications, skin sutures should usually be removed 7–10 days after surgery*
Under good healing conditions most surgical skin wounds heal after about 5–7 days, so the recommendation of removal after 7–10 days allows a few extra days to make sure the tissue is strong enough.

This would not necessarily be long enough in all situations. If there had been tension on the sutures, contamination by bacteria or animal interference with the wound, then the sutures might need to be left in place for longer.

3. A *In old nomenclature 2/0 suture material is one size thicker than 3/0*
The BPC gauges start with 10/0 as the finest material and increase in size to 2/0. 0 is the next size up, and the sizes then increase from 1 to 6.

The metric system is more logical. The number of the suture gives the diameter of the thread in mm multiplied by 10. Therefore 5 metric has a diameter of 0.5 mm.

There is no easy way to convert between the two systems, but two of the more commonly used sizes are 2/0 which is the equivalent of 3 metric, and 3/0 which is the same as 2 metric.

4. B *The horizontal mattress suture is an everting pattern*
This means that the wound edges have a tendency to
pucker up, and do not lie flat.

The other suture patterns: simple interrupted, cruciate
mattress and Ford interlocking suture patterns all produce
good wound edge apposition, with no inversion or
eversion.

5. A *0.2 metric is the smallest suture material*
In BPC gauge this is the same as 10/0.

6. C *The suture material which is monofilament is polypropylene
(Prolene)*
Silk, catgut and polyglactin 910 (Vicryl) are all braided
suture materials.

7. A *A curved cutting needle would appear triangular in cross
section, with the apex of the triangle on the inside of the curve*
The reverse cutting needle is similar except that the apex is
on the outside of the curve. Cutting needles are usually
used for skin and tough tissues.

The needle with a round cross section and fine tapered
point is described as round bodied, and is relatively
atraumatic.

8. A *Wire suture material is sized in Gauge, e.g. 20 g*
The numbers decrease as the wire gets thicker, so the
coarsest is 18 g, and the finest is 40 g.

Obstetrics and paediatrics

1. B *Oestrus can be prevented, suppressed or postponed by using progestagens*
Progestagens are drugs which mimic the effect of progesterone. Progesterone is produced during pregnancy by the corpus luteum, and acts to keep the uterus in the state needed to maintain the pregnancy. It also acts on the anterior pituitary to prevent the release of follicle stimulating hormone (FSH) and luteinizing hormone (LH). In the absence of FSH and LH the animal will not come into heat, and therefore will not ovulate. Using progestagens has the same effect.

2. B *The post-parturient condition that causes shivering, muscle spasm, collapse and disorientation in the lactating bitch is lactation tetani (eclampsia)*
Lactation tetani or eclampsia is caused by low blood calcium. The bitch produces so much milk that her readily available supplies of calcium are used up, and her blood levels fall. This results in failure of normal nerve and muscle function. Without rapid calcium supplementation the bitch could die, so these cases must be considered as medical emergencies. Intravenous calcium borogluconate should be given until the clinical signs start to resolve.

Metritis is inflammation of the uterus, usually caused by bacteria entering the uterus through the cervix during parturition. Mastitis is inflammation and infection of the mammary glands. Parvovirus infection in the adult animal causes vomiting and diarrhoea. However, if the bitch had been vaccinated it would not produce significant disease.

3. B *Neonates will not receive the full value of colostrum if it is given later than 36 hours after birth because they are unable to absorb the antibodies directly into the blood stream*
If an animal drinks colostrum shortly after birth, the antibodies in the colostrum are not digested as normal proteins would be, but are absorbed directly into the intestinal capillaries. These antibodies provide protection for the neonate against diseases that the mother has either been exposed to or been vaccinated against.

After 24–36 hours, the intestinal wall in the young animal changes, and the antibodies are no longer absorbed unchanged, but are digested in the same way as other proteins. The change in the intestinal wall is known as closure, and it is one of the main reasons that it is imperative for a neonate to receive an adequate supply of colostrum in the first few hours after birth.

4. C *Pups' and kittens' eyes open 10–14 days after birth*

5. D *None of the statements are true*
The queen is a seasonal breeder which means that there are only certain times of the year that she will come into season. The season starts in the spring and continues through to the autumn. She is polyoestrous, which means that during this time she will show several oestrous cycles, before entering anoestrus.

The queen is an induced ovulator so she will only ovulate once she has been mated. A queen that is not mated will therefore enter oestrus several times during a breeding season, but will not actually ovulate.

6. C *Uterine inertia is not a type of foetal dystocia*
Dystocias can be classified as maternal or foetal depending on the cause. Foetal dystocias arise either due to foetal oversize, an abnormal foetus, or some type of malpresentation. Maternal dystocias include uterine inertia, birth canal abnormalities, or some other physical obstruction.

7. B *The puerperium is the term used to describe the period after birth during which the uterus returns to normal*
The uterus usually takes between 4 to 6 weeks to involute or return to its normal size.

8. C *The hormone present through metoestrus in the bitch is progesterone*
Follicle stimulating hormone (FSH) is produced during proestrus and is the hormone that causes follicular maturation. As the follicles mature they release oestrogen, which increases in concentration until it peaks just prior to ovulation. The peak in oestrogen levels triggers a surge in luteinizing hormone (LH) which stimulates ovulation and the development of the corpus luteum. The LH surge occurs during oestrus.

The corpus luteum produces progesterone for several weeks after ovulation. This phase is metoestrus, after which the corpus luteum regresses and the bitch, if not pregnant, returns to anoestrus.

9. D *No drugs can be used in the event of a misalliance in the queen*
In the bitch oestrogen compounds such as oestrodiol benzoate can be used to terminate a misalliance and bring the animal back into oestrus providing they are given within four days of mating.

Oestrogens cannot be used in the queen as they are relatively toxic to cats and cause bone marrow suppression. The only options are either to allow the pregnancy to continue, or to spey the cat.

10. D *The average duration of oestrus in the bitch is 9 days*
The average timings for the stages of the oestrus cycle in the bitch are: proestrus 9 days, oestrus 9 days, metoestrus 50–60 days, anoestrus 4 months.

This gives a total oestrous cycle of 7 months. These are only average figures though, and individual animals can show wide variations from these timings.

11. D *A breech birth occurs when a foetus is delivered in posterior longitudinal presentation, dorsal position with hindlimbs flexed*
The terms presentation, position and posture can be used to accurately define the way a pup or kitten is delivered. A breech birth occurs when the pup is coming backwards, the right way up, but the legs are flexed so that it is trying to come out bottom first. Often these cannot be delivered easily, and assistance is required.

12. C *If an animal is primigravid it means that this is her first litter*
The term multigravid refers to an animal that has had one or more litters previously.
   Uniparous describes a species that normally only carries one foetus.

13. B *A week-old orphan pup being hand reared should be fed every four hours*
Up to one week of age it should be fed every two hours, but this can be decreased to every four hours at a week of age, providing the pup is growing well and putting on weight. Over the next two weeks the frequency of feeding can gradually be reduced to just four feeds a day. Once the pup reaches three weeks of age it is possible to start introducing solid foods as well as milk feeds.

14. D *Progesterone is tested for to determine whether a bitch is ready for mating or not*
Progesterone is only produced after ovulation has occurred and the corpus luteum has formed, and so it is the only reliable indicator of ovulation. The other hormones are present before and during oestrus, and so do not provide any indication of when to mate the bitch. If a bitch is mated within two days of ovulating the chances of conception are good.

15. D *If a vaginal smear was taken from a bitch during oestrus the predominant cells would be cornified cells*
An alternative method to blood testing is to use vaginal smears to determine when a bitch comes into oestrus.

In proestrus the main cell types are red blood cells and some round epithelial cells. As the bitch moves towards oestrus, the red blood cells decrease in numbers, and the epithelial cells becomes more crenated and do not have nuclei.

Smears taken in metoestrus show the presence of many white blood cells.

16. B *Strabismus is a squint*
This is seen as a normal finding in many kittens, and in most cases it resolves as they get older. However, many Siamese retain the squint throughout their lives.

17. A *Semen for Artificial Insemination (AI) is usually collected from the tom cat using electro-ejaculation*
In the dog the most usual methods are either digital manipulation or the use of an artificial vagina.

18. D *Vaginal smears can be stained using Leishman's, Wright's or Difquik stains*
Any of the Romanowsky stains can be used for staining vaginal smears. Romanowsky stains contain two dyes, a blue dye which stains alkaline areas, and a red dye which has an affinity for acidic areas within cells. In this way different types of cells can be readily identified.

19. C *The ferret is an induced ovulator*
As well as the ferret, the cat and the rabbit are induced ovulators. Most other small animal species are spontaneous ovulators.

20. B *Palpation can be used as a method of pregnancy diagnosis after 3–4 weeks of the pregnancy*
At this stage the foetuses are just detectable as small swellings within the uterus. Individual parts of the foetuses cannot be distinguished until they are about 6–7 weeks old.

It is not possible to accurately tell the number of foetuses through palpation.